KINGDOM IN THE SKY

KINGDOM IN THE SKY

by

John S. Cunningham

SOUVENIR PRESS

First published 1975 by Souvenir Press, Ltd.,
95 Mortimer Street, London WIN 8HP
and simultaneously in Canada by
J. M. Dent & Sons (Canada) Ltd,
Ontario, Canada

ISBN 0 285 62097 5

Printed and bound in Great Britain
by Tinlings (1973) Limited, Prescot, Merseyside
(a member of the Oxley Printing Group Ltd.)

Dedicated to my wife Penny and to all the members of the Britain-Nepal Medical Trust, past and present.

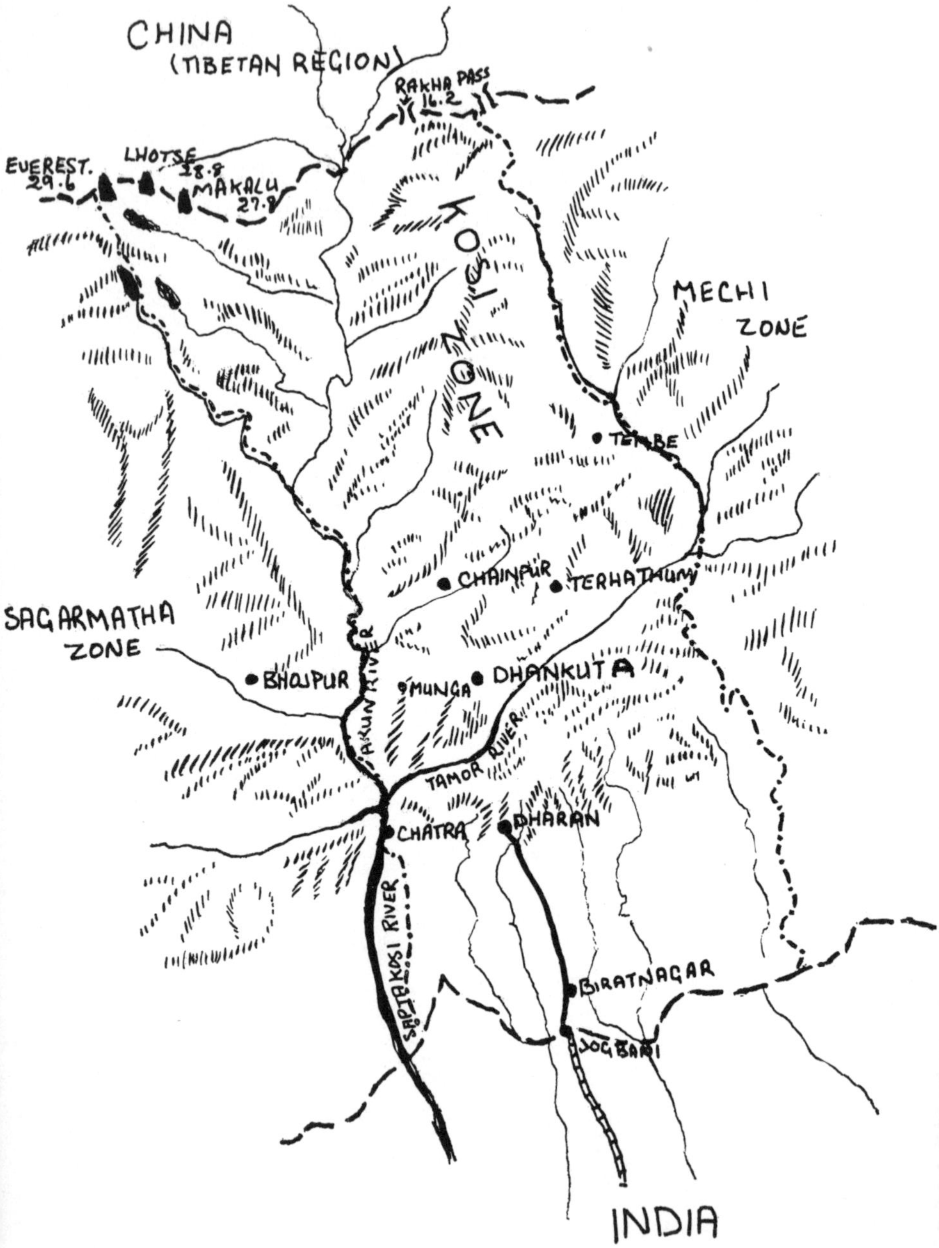

SKETCH MAP OF KOSI ZONE, EAST NEPAL

Contents

List of Illustrations

Foreword

Nepal is one of the most fascinating countries in the world. The pattern of daily life there has remained almost unchanged for many centuries, and we can still perceive in the remote villages of this mountainous land the ancient virtues of family and community life, where people subsist on the soil. The rat race of competitive commerce and careerism, divisive ambitions for material and social advancement, have so far made little or no impact on the pattern of existence in Nepal.

Perhaps for this very reason, the first inescapable impression of all visitors is of the happiness of its people. The smiling gaiety of the Nepalis was first commented upon way back in 1843 by Henry Lawrence, British Resident in Kathmandu. He arrived not many years after the British had invaded Nepal in the days of the East India Company, and sampled the courage of its warriors, who were soon to join the ranks of the Company's forces and become known as Gurkhas. Gaiety and courage are the hallmarks of the Nepalese people.

But no one who travels in the remoter parts of the country can fail also to be moved by the physical suffering which the villagers patiently endure for lack of medical services: pain is a concomitant of isolation from the developed world beyond the mountains. It was to alleviate this suffering that John and Penny Cunningham conceived their imaginative enterprise of an independent mission to Nepal, which has made such a significant contribution towards improving health in eastern Nepal during the past six years. Spurning the official channels for aid programmes and without seeking government financial backing, John Cunningham succeeded in gaining acceptance of his offer of private medical assistance, largely through his own enthusiasm and sincerity. The mission launched by the Britain-Nepal Medical Trust was essentially an adventure by a splendid little band of pioneers, inspired by the knowledge that there was a real need to be met in a country where, despite or because of the grandeur of its scenery, life is hard.

I am the more happy to write a foreword to this delightful account of their life and work in Nepal for the fact that, like the author, I love its people, and because one of the original team was my daughter.

JOHN HUNT

CHAPTER I

An Idea is Born

'And all my fortunes at thy foot I'll lay
And follow thee my lord throughout the world.'

ROMEO AND JULIET

In 1962 I had been qualified as a doctor for one year and was working as a House Physician to the Children's department of St Thomas's Hospital. At the time I was well aware of a particular medical student working with us; but I did not know that she was to be my wife, nor did I know in what direction my career in medicine would take me.

After my six months at St Thomas's, I found a post as ship's doctor on a passenger liner sailing to Africa. After the rigours of hospital life, I did little medicine, made a number of friends, saw a great deal of a country that had always appealed to me, and found my appetite for travelling whetted. But I returned home, accepted a position as a Registrar in a South London hospital, and renewed my association with the St Thomas's Hospital Bar. Penny was by then taking her final exams. A five-shilling bet found four of us in an expensive night-club in the West End drinking brandy cocktails at twelve-and-six a time. A year later saw a considerable fall in my bank balance and on June 18th 1966, we were married in Farnham.

After a honeymoon in Spain, we returned to our new home in Blackheath, without any clear plans for the future.

Both Penny and I had known from an early age that we wanted to practise medicine, though neither of our families provided us with any particular medical background. Penny's father was a solicitor with his home in Surrey, and my father had worked for the Imperial Tobacco Company — an even more unlikely starting point for a medical career. Penny, the eldest of three girls, had been educated at Godolphin School, Salisbury, from where she went to St Thomas's; and I had my schooling at Clifton College, Bristol, after which I spent three years at Cambridge.

When I was ten, I had spent an uncomfortable seven weeks in the Bristol Royal Infirmary with acute nephritis (a kidney disease) and I have no doubt that this was the reason for my decision to take up a medical career. From that time onwards, various people helped me to achieve my goal, not the least of them the master at Clifton who told me (in no uncertain terms) that I was to go to Cambridge, an idea which had never till then crossed my mind. This was to impose a further financial burden on my parents, who had already invested considerably in my schooling.

Now we had decisions to make; and it soon became apparent that neither of us would be able to settle until I had seen more of the world and achieved my ambition of doing something of value in some part of the earth where my medical skills were most urgently required. I wanted to get away from the limited medicine I had been practising as a Hospital Registrar for three years, with a predictable future already mapped out before me. We both rebelled against so restricted a use of a training in which not only we but others had invested so much; I suppose we wanted in some sense to give back a little of the privilege we felt we had received. The decision was perhaps more difficult for Penny, who certainly did not lightly give up the security of our home; but she was far-seeing enough to realise that our future happiness depended upon our doing something bold and imaginative now.

How then could we use our qualifications most meaningfully? We knew that doctors were in short supply throughout the world. So we went to Governmental organisations for advice, but they had nothing to offer us. We were on our own. Yet there were others like us. Many of our friends found themselves in a similar position — unwilling to commit themselves to a particular field in medicine and yet unable to decide on an alternative — and it occurred to us that we might establish our own team and offer ourselves to some organisation which could make use of our services in an area of the world medically less well endowed than our own. We had no idea more concrete than that.

So we sat down with some statistics on world-wide medical facilities. Nigeria appeared to be the most in need, with the lowest doctor/patient ratio in the world. Nepal came next. Nepal was immediately appealing, conjuring up pictures of Everest and Annapurna, of pagodas and temples. So I went to see the Ministry of Overseas Development. It seemed that the Ministry could use us only if an official request for assisance were made by His Majesty's Government of Nepal. But since His Majesty's Government was at that time entirely unaware that anyone from Britain wished to come to Nepal to practise medicine, the chance of such a request being made did not seem very great.

The idea would not die, however. Two hundred doctors for eleven million people, we argued — they *must* welcome help. So following a decision reached in a haze of beer funes and cigarette smoke on September 20th 1966, we drafted a letter to the Director of Health Services, Kathmandu, asking whether he would be interested in receiving a team of doctors and nurses from the United Kingdom, who would be willing to work in Nepal for a non-specified period of time. We sent similar enquiries at the same time to the Health Services in Assam and Iran.

I have often been asked since: why, among all the countries that needed medical help, choose Nepal? And I am still not certain that I can answer the question clearly. I guess we were attracted in the first place by the same romantic image that attracts the hippies, the young from all over the world: the image of the remote mountain vastness, land of myth and legend, where history goes back into a dim mysterious past, both wise and innocent, yet where time stands still: a sort of Shangri-la. We knew little concrete about the place. But we were excited by the idea of it.

Almost immediately, a reply came back from Nepal. When I look back on it now, it was something of a miracle. We merely wrote a letter to the Ministry of Health in Kathmandu. Had we written this letter to fifty other Governments we would probably not have got a single reply. We were being supremely optimistic. And yet there was a young doctor in the Nepal Department of Health who saw our letter, thought it was interesting and went to the trouble of replying. We got to know him pretty well as a friend when we eventually went to Nepal, but it was really a piece of extraordinary luck that he noticed our letter at all.

Our response, which was also prompt, indicated that we would like to provide a mobile surgical/medical team, comprising six to eight doctors and nurses, who would be used as the Government of Nepal wished. It can now be said that this offer was a piece of amazing cheek, as the team consisted only of Penny and myself and the preparations and finances were still pipe-dreams.

However, we were elated because our assumptions had been proved correct, someone really did want us, and the least we could do, we felt, was to make a determined effort to provide the services required.

To carry out our project there were three main requirements — a team, adequate finance and equipment.

We realised also that our knowledge of Nepal was sadly limited and we immediately set out to improve it by buying maps and books, ransacking local libraries and generally making contact with as many people as possible who knew about the Himalayan Kingdom. As our knowledge and enthusiasm grew, our field of conversation grew smaller until we became extraordinary bores. However, our friends did not desert us but gradually accepted that we really were in earnest.

Our first recruit to the team was Barney Rosedale, unmarried and a contemporary of Penny at Thomas's. I first mentioned the subject of Nepal to him when he was about to leave England for a year in Nigeria. 'What a marvellous idea, I'd love to come,' was his immediate response. 'When I get back from Ibadan I'll be there.' He included himself in the project as if it were the simplest thing in the world! Thin and wiry, he soon proved a person with tremendous ideas and terrific energy. So fast indeed did his ideas occur that he often infuriated me because I couldn't keep pace — in Nepal he would always be striding north into the hills or vanishing into India endowed with an enthusiasm which left most of us shaking our heads in amazement. It was he who was eventually to take over from me as team leader — he is the sort of person who will always be wanted and always be there, and as I write he is 22,000 feet up Everest with Chris Bonnington!

Even in that first year, he bombarded us with letters from Nigeria, making suggestions, and sparking off ideas, because he of all our team members could see ahead, both the potentialities and the enormous difficulties in our scheme.

Even before he left he had us deep in books on drains, latrines, explosives and buildings; Army manuals indicating how deep we should have our sanitation pit; tomes on how to build mud walls in a monsoon, how to be electricians, plumbers, engineers, with hardly a hint of medicine. He had done his National Service as a sapper, and kept pointing out that we were going to have to be 'Jacks of all trades' so we might as well start now. How true his words were to prove!

Just before he left for Nigeria he introduced us to our next recruit, John Ward, a surgeon trained at St Mary's, currently working at St George's. He had wide knowledge of general surgery and in the special fields of genito-urinary and plastic surgery, and he was enthusiastic about the prospect of widening his surgical experience. With some difficulty he was able to obtain leave of absence from his hospital appointment to join us, and set about approaching commercial companies for the supplies he would need. A cottage he had recently bought in Dorset became a useful rendezvous for all us. He was to fall in love with the beautiful blonde Sheena, one of our team nurses, and the two of them were eventually married in Kathmandu.

Then came Rosemary Reid, a Middlesex-trained nurse, daughter of a country doctor, who happened to be completing her midwifery training at Beckenham, so she spent a lot of time with us in Blackheath helping to stem the rising tide of correspondence. She was a redhead with the proverbial temper and an immediate emotional responsiveness to go with it. She was to find that her physical and emotional sensitivity made her very vulnerable in Nepal — the heat and the humidity affected her more than the rest of us, and her midwifery involved her with some of the most tragic of the cases with which we had to deal, for any mother coming into hospital to have a baby tended to be there because she was already seriously ill with anaemia, or because there was a serious birth complication. Rosemary was often surrounded with death and misery, and she suffered, brave and hardworking as she tried to be.

Through Rosemary we met Gill Kellie, also Middlesex-trained, who was working at Kingston in Casualty and Theatre. Small, bustling, attractive, she was to prove one of the mainstays of the team. She was independent and could organise, and she threw herself into everything. She was as much at home on a horse as behind the wheel of a landrover, and had nerves of steel — since she travelled with Barney on the trip out, these came in useful from the beginning. Yet her outer toughness only half concealed a great inner kindliness, which suited her marvellously to the work in Nepal, and helped her to get on well with the Nepali staff.

Suddenly we had the nucleus of our team. Penny and I at this time were keeping body and soul together by working in Locum General Practice, while Penny was also completing a Family Planning course and doing occasional Anaesthetic sessions. We began to feel as though our project, a vision for so long, was at last an almost concrete reality.

In our quest for further knowledge we joined the Britain-Nepal Society. This society has its base in London and comprises nearly 400 members, men and women who have affiliations of various kinds with Nepal; mountaineers and diplomats, Gurkhas and botanists. One of the first things we learned was the compelling hold that Nepal seems to have over everyone who has spent time there. And through this society came a further recruit for our team — Lord Hunt's daughter Prue, a recently qualified nurse and the second youngest member of the team. She had the spirit of adventure in her, like her father, and had always wanted to see Nepal.

Vint Chadwick came to us through John. He was a recently qualified physician, stocky, capable, reliable, with a dry sense of humour which was often to rescue our spirits in times of difficulty. We expected to need a pathologist, so he managed to get a six-months' appointment at St George's Pathology department. Not long before we left for Nepal he married Di — we all went to their wedding in Hertfordshire. Di was also a fully qualified nurse, very vivacious and full of fun, who bore her subsequent hardships as well as anyone, though I suspect that, rather like Penny, she would really have preferred to settle down quietly at home and have children!

Peter Hawksworth was the youngest member of the team. Only nineteen, he had recently lost his father, who had been a surgeon. He had no idea what he wanted to do with his life, but he wanted a break from England, and he had a flair for mechanics. He was thin as a rake when we first met him, but persevering to the point of doggedness, and he threw himself gladly into his work and indeed without his efforts we might never have left England!

CHAPTER II

We Equip Ourselves

Who were we? We eventually decided to call ourselves the Britain-Nepal Medical Expedition. It certainly sounded impressive. With our team assembled, we now had to begin to equip ourselves.

Pharmaceutical companies seemed to be the obvious first line of approach. These companies give away thousands of pounds worth of samples daily — surely our project was deserving of some support? With our slightly pompous title, an ancient typewriter and a piece of paper on which we had set out our — at that time — somewhat vague aims and intentions, we wrote what seemed like millions of letters of request.

I must stress the extreme generosity of some of these companies — whom we were compelled to bother over and over again. Why they should have thought us any more worthy of support than the hundreds of others whose appeals they received, I do not know, but something unusual in our letter struck the imagination of one Managing Director, who telephoned me to say that he would like to discuss the project further, and his help and advice took us on, amazingly, to the next stage.

Every day, he pointed out, firms in this country receive in the post appeals for money and equipment, and some companies have a whole department just to deal with this correspondence. (Some of the letters that I saw myself when I visited industrial concerns have to be seen to be believed: a school team intending to camp in North Wales for one week requires all its groceries; a garden fête requires containers for jam and marmalade). Certain companies have had to stop the donation of free products altogether. So our adviser recommended us from the start to be precise in what we proposed to do and to present our plans as concretely as possible; to obtain patronage from other professional people; and to involve our patrons both as advisers and active supporters. We were lucky to receive such good advice, and we shall not forget this, nor those companies who helped us right from those early stages, before we had anything except our sheet of paper.

Our flat in Blackheath began to disintegrate — the small hall became a storeroom and our dining room became an office. Giving a dinner party became a major removal problem. The sitting room was fast becoming a sea of paper. The postman thought we had become part of a mail order business, and it was soon apparent that unless we found storage space we might have to move out altogether.

Again help was at hand and the Managing Director of a well-known packing company gave us the use of a bay in a warehouse in South-east London to store our rapidly growing mound of equipment. Two years previously the same warehouse had been involved with the packing of all the equipment for an expedition to climb Makalu. Little did we know then that in less than two years we would be able to stand on our roof in Nepal and see this very same peak soaring into the sky away to the north.

Letter-writing trebled. We tried never to duplicate letters, but to write individual letters to each company, preferably addressed in person to the Managing Director. Trade Directories and Stock Exchange Gazettes became part of our library. We soon knew the names of the Chairmen of companies we had never known existed. The *Daily Telegraph* Information Service supplied the answers to hundreds of questions — was X a substitute for Y? Was A owned by an American Company or a German one? Did B produce high-voltage cable?

Personally addressed letters undoubtedly produced dividends. In two years we were to write nearly 10,000, and we are still writing them today. Some then unknown people are now our firm personal friends. Others are sick to death of hearing from us. Thirty percent of the people we approached ignored us; ten percent responded with stereotyped letters saying that they were unable to help; a further fifty percent said no, but wished us luck; and ten percent gave us the help we so desperately needed. They offered equipment and pharmaceutical supplies to start with, then the occasional financial donation.

We opened a bank account, and my own bank manager made the first contribution. I think that his motive at the time may well have been simply the pleasure of seeing an account in my name with a positive balance. But things were looking brighter every minute.

We turned from pharmaceutical companies (sixty-five of them), only two of whom contributed nothing, to companies manufacturing medical and surgical equipment; from them to the giants of industry. Every day brought a deluge through the letter-box, almost like Christmas — and just as at Christmas, thank-you letters had to be written.

By April 1967 our warehouse was beginning to look like a department store. Books and baked beans, sutures and soap lay all around. We worked like beavers trying to catalogue the non-stop flow of donations. The financial side was improving daily.

Correspondence with our Embassy in Kathmandu was regular, but the Nepalese Government would not come to any decision as to where our team could be used. It was suggested that I should go to Kathmandu to initiate personal talks with His Majesty's Goverment and to gain some first-hand knowledge of the kind of conditions we could expect to encounter.

CHAPTER III

First Glimpse of Nepal

I left London Airport on April 14th 1967 in a Spring temperature of fifty degrees, and in twelve hours I was in Delhi. The temperature had risen nearly forty degrees and within minutes my temper was rising at about the same rate. This was to be my first of many experiences with officialdom in India, which now merely make me laugh and shrug my shoulders, but at the time drove me into a frenzy of impotence and anger.

I was travelling on a joint passport at the time, a mistake which involved me in almost fifteen minutes of futile explanation that my wife was really not with me; and I lived to regret the frivilous suggestion that Penny was probably in my suitcase, because it was taken quite seriously. Several degrees hotter, I won through this barrier to be met immediately by another. My plane to Kathmandu had been delayed until the following day. I was, however, given a card with my new booking and departure time.

Fortunately I was able to stay with friends in Delhi — Sally, whom I had first met as a nurse at St Thomas', and her husband David — and the following day, now a little more adapted to eastern habits, I was back at the airport, this time to find that the plane had left an our earlier than usual for Kathmandu as the pilot had to be back for the departure of a senior Government official on a state visit. I had a feeling that Kathmandu was holding out on me.

The following day we climbed at last into a dust-laden

sky and turned away eastward over Bihar. Below me was one huge dustbowl — Bihar had had no rain for two years, thousands were dying of hunger or thirst. Then, suddenly, leaving the dust and the dying behind, we turned north over the forest area of Nepal, the Terai: jungle and swamps, rivers and paddi fields, until recently a death-trap to all Europeans and inhabited only by the Tharu tribe whose origin is still obscure.

From the Terai into the foothills and away to the north lies one of the most magnificent views in the world. A solid wall of ice and snow stretches as far as the eye can see, from Kashmir in the west to West Bengal and Sikkim in the east, pierced occasionally by high passes which supply the trade routes between Tibet and Nepal.

Then in twenty minutes we were dropping into the lush and fertile Kathmandu valley.

As my plane circled over Kathmandu I looked down for the first time on the temples and the riot of life and colour which my imagination had pictured for so long. I was not at first disappointed. We had no sooner landed at the airport than I was surrounded by a clamour of children demanding in broken English whether or not I required a taxi. That was my first impression of Kathmandu: no orderly taxi queue like at Waterloo Station, just a general hubbub and a feeling of rush and hurry and complete disorganisation. Cheerful, laughing, I wasn't quite sure which way to turn. Then as I drove the three miles to the British Embassy I was struck by the smell of the streets: a hint of curry; a hint of dust; a gentle bustle but no real rush as the side road from the airport narrows down into the town itself. I was amazed by the size of the vegetables piled outside the shops: enormous turnips, cabbages and cauliflowers: and by the sight of the cows walking down the street as if they had as much right to space there as the people. Cows and people looked sleek and well-fed, in comfortable contrast to the misery of Bihar.

On the way in, one sees, however, little of the really old part of Kathmandu, little of the temples which are all situated in the Bazaar itself in the centre of the town. Instead one sees hotels sprung up for the benefit of the tourist, and little different from the hotels outside any modern city in the world. It was not until much later that I was able to go into the back streets and find a world to measure against my fantasies.

That was 1966, before the world had discovered Kathmandu; before the hippies had come, and the aid schemes, and the foreign companies. It was only to be two years before I returned, but during that time Embassies and Legations had increased fourfold, and everywhere you went you saw the influence of the Western world. In 1966, however, there were few European faces, all of which tended to turn up at the same social gatherings. But the town was lively enough, with screaming voices and honking horns and rattling cars.

Driving in Nepal is always a hazardous business. The taxi drivers, like those in India, tend to put the fear of God into everyone, and when I drove in a taxi I always remembered the little story of the Pope and the Archbishop of Canterbury waiting to be allowed through the Gates of Heaven. They had been sitting there for a number of months and still St Peter was saying 'I am sorry but I cannot allow you in', when a little man in a dirty white coat came up the stairs, knocked on the gates and was immediately allowed through. The Pope and the Archbishop of Canterbury, being a trifle put out by the incident, asked St Peter why he had been let in and they had not. 'It is quite simple,' replied the Saint, 'He was a taxi driver in Calcutta and he put the fear of God into more people than the two of you put together.'

I settled down to discuss our problems with members of the British Embassy, and their careful briefing at once convinced me that, although our services might be welcomed, we were still a long way from any decision, let alone any form of contract. It was eventually decided that I should approach Her Royal Highness Princess Princep Shah, His

Majesty King Mahendra's sister-in-law, and request her support as Chairman of the Nepalese Red Cross, under whose auspices we might be employed. This I did and was much impressed by her affection for our country and her great courtesy. She agreed to be our Patron and discussed various possibilities as to where our team could be of most value.

It seemed likely that we would be in most demand in the hill areas, especially in Western Nepal, which had very few doctors. So during my last week it was decided that I should fly over to the west, have a look at the country and try to appreciate some of the problems with which we would be presented.

The town of Pokhara is about one hundred and fifty miles due west of Kathmandu, and one morning I found myself flying over the mountains and down into a valley which lies at an altitude of only two thousand feet and commands one of the most beautiful views in the world. As you circle into the valley you look up at the enormous mountain faces of Annapurna, Dhaulagiri and Macchapuchare. The first thing that struck me about the town was the almost total absence of vehicles; there were just one or two dilapidated landrovers which had been carried in over the hills. The centre of the main street was lined with paving stones, and mules, beautifully decorated with coloured head dresses and laden with rice, blocked your way.

In Pokhara I found myself a tiny little Tibetan hotel and settled down for the night, basking in the coolness of the evening, and watching the sun drop behind the mountains. The following day I arranged a porter and set off for the hills. The porter spoke very little English and I, at that time, spoke no Nepali, but somehow we managed with a fair amount of sign language to get on together and travel in the right direction.

The prosperity I had noted in Kathamndu had seemed already to be missing in Pokhara and as we headed north through the tiny villages, I began to realise that I was leaving civilisation behind. I was coming to the point where I was at last seeing the bare face of Nepal; but a week was by no means long enough for me to see very much of Western Nepal, and it was with regret that I had to return to the capital.

Although strongly advised to wait in Kathmandu for a final dicision, I had been away one month already and felt I could not afford to stay any longer, either financially or in view of the increasing work at home. So it was decided that the Embassy would continue to negotiate on our behalf. But if this short visit — although inconclusive — had not been made, I am quite certain that we would never have got to Nepal.

CHAPTER IV

Departure

On the plane home, facing two Qantas breakfasts (in Teheran and Athens) and one lunch at 7.45 a.m. over Zurich, I considered our position.

Nepal needed our services, of that there was no doubt. But Nepal is a proud country, she courts aid only on her own terms, and we could not afford to make demands. We would have to wait patiently, offer suggestions and accept whatever decision His Majesty's Government might eventually make.

On my return it was decided, on the advice of our Patrons, that the Britain-Nepal Medical Expedition must become a Registered Charity. This step we have never regretted. We were after all not really an expedition: going overland to Kathmandu had been done many times before — with a little preparation, it amounts to no more than driving to Edinburgh and back eight times — and the main purpose of the venture was not to travel, but to establish something permanent, something of real value to Nepal.

The formalities required to become a charity are many and various. They are also extremely frustrating. At one point we reached an impasse, when the Bank of England would not give us the required permission unless His Majesty's Income Tax Inspectors gave theirs, and the tax department would grant permission only if the Bank would.

But in July 1967 all was signed and sealed, and we were now the Britain-Nepal Medical Trust Limited.

Our terms of reference were defined, our principal obligation being to supply medical aid in the form of personnel and equipment to developing countries, in the first place to Nepal. The cost of such aid would be attributable to the Trust. We were also committed to undertaking medical research of value to the Nepalese and to world health in general.

Once we were registered as a charity, the response to our appeal improved greatly. Industrial companies, public and private charities, and individuals were all interested. Coffee parties, wine and cheese parties added to the funds and our bank balance improved so much that we were able to think about spending some of it.

Inevitably we chose landrovers as our means of transport. Barney provided his own short wheel-base, and we ordered two long wheel-bases from the Rover company. John and I went on the landrover maintenance course and within a few weeks we were the proud owners of two gleaming white trucks.

From Solihull the vehicles went to Sussex, where Pilchers adapted them for use as mobile surgeries. Cupboards were fitted, a water filtration unit, even a hand-basin with running water; and kerosene tanks, spare petrol and water tanks, and locked safety compartments were incorporated. We tried the ingenuity of this firm to the limit, but they made no complaint, and the result was excellent.

Time ticked by with still no word from Nepal. We booked air passages for April 18th for the vehicles and team from Southend to Calais, still uncertain whether the project would come off at all.

But March 20th brought the decision at last. A cable from our Embassy in Kathmandu to the Foreign Office in London stated that His Majesty's Government requested us to come to Nepal to work in Biratnagar in the south-east of Nepal. Hastily-studied maps showed Biratnagar to be about as far away from our prospective zone as possible; and we were deeply disappointed that we were not going to the hills. Once more we sat round and agonised over endless cups of coffee; but we were at least welcomed and wanted, and no-one felt we could refuse to go. In the end, we were to find that Biratnagar had been a wise choice after all.

Last-minute preparations were now put under way. We sent ten tons of donations by sea to Calcutta — from food to footwear, from stainless steel to stethoscopes, from diaries to drugs. We bought tents and sleeping bags, had passport photographs and chest X-rays taken, and a massive series of vaccinations. Days were too short; flats had to be rented, powers of attorney given, insurance obtained. Exhausted but enthusiastic we set off to Henley-on-Thames for a 'trial run'. It was a frustrating moment when we found how badly we had miscalculated our load — the mound of equipment simply would not fit into the Rovers. Out went the excess to go by sea. A cold night proved that 'mountain tents' sweated and that survival sheets produced enough condensation to drown in.

As the team collected in the field behind Prue's father's house on the day before our departure, with three landrovers and mounds of equipment scattered all over the place, my immediate impression was one of utter chaos. As I watched everybody going about their jobs, it seemed to me impossible that within a few days all eleven of us would be crossing the continent heading for the East. Vint took one look at the situation and said something to the effect that 'with all this bloody lot we'll never even get as far as Dover'.

Tempers were a little frayed. There seemed to be so much to do and so short a time in which to do it. A signwriter was hastily procured from Oxford, and he sat on his stool in the middle of the field painting the Nepal flag and the Union Jack on the sides of each car. The large tent proved difficult to erect and suddenly we remembered we had forgotten the mosquito netting. Peter tore off to find some, and then of course came the problem of stitching it on to the tent. I think by the end of the evening when we were all tired, we inwardly thought we would never get going at all, and the night itself didn't help. It was very cold indeed, we all slept badly and woke in the morning rather dejected, but enthusiasm soon strengthened again, and, each one of us taking a proportion of the work, chaos was turned into a semblance of order.

As the Press reporters arrived to photograph our departure, we looked back over the anxieties and frustrations of the previous fifteen months and wondered what the future held for each of us. We had really been extraordinarily lucky, in spite of the many setbacks. Whenever we had felt truly despondent, thinking we would never raise all the money and equipment we required, suddenly out of the blue the morning post, or an unexpected telephone call, had somehow brought us what we needed. And almost on the eve of our departure a big Trust had found us a windfall of £10,000 (then in India, but available for transfer to Nepal) which was to make all the difference in the world to our early months.

Eventually all the cars were packed, final farewells made and we set off in convoy for Southend.

CHAPTER V

The Journey — Europe

In case anyone should wonder why we went overland, the decision was purely and simply a matter of expense: just over £600 enabled three vehicles and eleven people to reach Kathmandu. By sea it would have cost over £2000 and taken just as long.

British United Airways landed us in France in twenty minutes, then our gleaming landrovers were photographed by Pressmen yet again. We remembered to drive off on the right hand side of the road and set off in convoy for the Franco-Belgian frontier.

We took the fastest route through Europe via Brussels and then by Autobahn to Munich, staying at recognised camping sites. But already we were finding that three vehicles and eleven people add up to a large number of problems. Convoy driving proved totally unsuitable, so we adopted a system of two-hourly stops, when the leading car pulled into a suitable lay-by and waited for the others to come up. Setting up and breaking camp was a headache and although we soon established a routine we very rarely managed either in less than an hour, which can prove very trying at the end of a long day's driving. Cooking was done by the girls and washing-up by the men on a rotating basis. We frowned on excessive use of cooking pots and utensils, and a congealed mass of cold porridge in a saucepan could easily provoke as much wrath as sources of animal protein in one's salad.

Nevertheless, our progress through Europe was fast; we adapted to each other's habits and tried to make our journey as comfortable as possible.

All of us enjoyed the beauty of the Bavarian Alps, and John brought out his new ciné camera, recently purchased in Munich. But once out of the mountains we came upon our first major problem: that of finding an apparently straightforward camping site marked on the A.A. carnet. The cars had been separated for more than an hour and each independently decided to make directly for the site. Barney found the site first, and after an hour waiting for John and me, decided he was in the wrong place. I arrived just after he had left and decided to return to the main road to find John. With no sign of him, I left a cryptic note on a signpost for him, which was actually found by Barney on his second time round. More by luck than by judgment, we found ourselves together again beside Lake Faunsee, where Vint and I had been doing some desultory fishing while waiting for the others. After this I tended to treat the camping guide only as a general direction-finder.

We were sorry to leave the Alps behind and even sorrier to reach the Zagreb-Belgrade motorway. For 300 miles this road runs flat and straight with almost no traffic through featureless countryside. The sight of one of our cars weaving all over the road, with the driver half asleep, made us reduce our two-hourly changes to only one.

From the rather drab and sombre cities of Yugoslavia we crossed the Dragoman pass into Bulgaria, the road cutting through wild and beautiful pine forests. The camping guide to Bulgaria showed several well equipped sites along this route, all of which proved to be non-existent, so our first night saw us pitching tents in a rather grubby apple orchard outside Sophia. The only evidence of the advertised swimming pool and showers was a small slab of concrete and a single cold tap, which produced an occasional air-locked gurgle of water. But we spent the evening in very congenial company at the local restaurant, drinking a Bulgarian wine which had the consistency and taste of blackcurrant syrup. We discussed England and the last war, clothes and customs, and avoided politics.

Throughout Bulgaria the iron curtain hangs over one like a shroud. The austere communal farms, drab way of life, furtive glances in the street, all tend to make one feel uncomfortable. The police practice of hiding in ditches and behind trees with walkie-talkie sets and then leaping out to fine one on the spot for some minor traffic transgression is particularly unnerving; and the hundred yards of scorched earth at the border, heavily wired and pill-boxed, even more so. We were glad to cross into Turkey.

The Turkish border town of Edirne held a pleasant surprise for us; the most efficient camping site I had ever seen, including showers, cooking rings, and even electric irons. We stayed for two days cleaning our clothes, our vehicles and ourselves. Already we had begun to appreciate some of the simpler amenities that we normally take for granted. Barney and Gill went off that night to sample the local hospitality, which proved excellent, judging by the condition of a rather crushed garbage can attached to the rear of their landrover the following morning.

Welcoming the slow-down in our headlong progress towards Asia, we turned into Greece and headed for the Aegean Sea and Alexandropolis, where we stayed for two days, Barney giving us graphic descriptions of his previous holidays in the Greek Islands. Two thousand years and more ago this area panted to the strain of marching soldiers, battles raged on land and sea, and the might of Greece stretched across the world. But today the people are very poor, their existence a day-to-day affair, and their comforts few. We spent our time lounging on the rocky beach and emptying our cupboards of a congealed mass of marmite and sugar. One evening we all went out to eat in Alexandropolis. It was an unmemorable meal until John decided to exercise his Greek by ordering a liqueur. To our consternation an enormous slab of chocolate cake was produced on a silver tray, so after this John wisely returned to the use of his own language.

Istanbul, the gateway to Asia, attracted some of us and

repelled others. Its Byzantine walls, thirty feet thick and equally high, had held for centuries against assault, and still dominate the entrance to the city. Today one brushes shoulders with Turks, Arabs, Germans and Americans. The Bazaars glitter with bronze and silver, with carpets and shawls. The noise is deafening, traffic regulations non-existent, the smell a cross between burning rubber and a sewage farm.

We toured the Bazaars with hands in our pockets, constantly endeavouring to save our women folk from the pinching fingers of an apparently sex-starved populace. We visited the Blue Mosque, of course, and admired its magnificent architecture. We saw jewel-encrusted swords and rooms full of Chinese porcelain. We drove our cars across the Golden Horn, and then crossed by ferry into Asia, 1800 miles and ten days from London.

CHAPTER VI

The Journey—Asia

The road to Ankara is wide and fast across barren countryside punctuated by small villages mostly built of mud and clay. On this road we found competition which was only to be surpassed in Iran. Twenty-ton lorries hurtled along at seventy miles per hour, mostly in the middle of the road. Attempts to overtake were greeted with rude gestures and immediate acceleration. No one seemed to care if you overtook on the left or the right, and on some occasions we actually had to take to the fields to avoid otherwise inevitable collision.

Ankara promised us another camping site. If it existed, we certainly never found it, and much to the amusement of the local people, we found ourselves encamped on the edge of the main highway trying hard to forget the smell of diesel fumes.

The carburettor on Barney's car was giving trouble and the exhaust manifolds on the other vehicles were constantly loosening, so we took the opportunity to go to the landrover dealers to see if matters could be improved. Whilst the cars were being examined a few of us went to the Embassy to pick up mail and arrange forwarding addresses.

There we had news of a much more serious problem. A cholera outbreak in Afghanistan had led to the closure of borders between that country and Iran and also possibly between Iran and Turkey. The Embassy very kindly launched an all-out assault on the local Health Ministry to gather up-to-date information, and telephoned the border posts direct. By mid-afternoon our landrovers were repaired, the Turco-Iranian frontier was declared open and we left the sun-baked streets of the capital to set out north towards the Black Sea, the Turkish Riviera.

By now much of our time was spent in searching for camping spots where we could hope for a little privacy. Everywhere we went the inquisitive instincts of the natives were aroused, and the cars were surrounded by hordes of children jabbering away in a language of which we knew not a word. Eventually we chose a sandy cove, well surrounded by rocky cliffs. The only entrance was down a narrow path in the middle of which was a massive boulder. Throwing caution to the winds, we inched by on the outside of the obstruction, trying to ignore the precipitous drop to the beach below, which would have ruined our vehicles and ourselves as well.

Camping on sand produces its own brand of discomfort, but we had our privacy at last and an air of calm prevailed as the setting sun coloured the sea deep purple. The silence was short-lived. Potential swimmers found the sea like — well, the proverbial monkey. I have never known sea so cold. Only four members of the party managed to get their knees wet. Little wonder that the coast was virtually deserted.

Away from the sea the weather became hotter, the countryside more like a desert, and camel trains became a familiar feature. The camels' haughty expressions and unerring spitting accuracy never ceased to amuse us!

We crossed another border to Tabriz, famous for its carpets. We didn't see a single carpet, but we did find the town a very suitable centre to replenish our stores, and then went on to Teheran, where we found our last official camp site, Gol-e-Sara, owned by a very pleasant couple who made us feel very much at home. We fell upon the cold showers like wolves on their prey and devoured quantities of iced coca-cola and lemon. This haven seemed to be the generally recognised stopping place of most overlanders. A visitors' book gave us some useful information as to whom and what to avoid in Teheran.

Teheran is a large bustling capital. Crossing the road is an attempt at suicide and driving the cars was an experience few wanted to repeat. No quarter is given and none expected. That we emerged unscathed is a miracle.

Penny, Sheena, John and I, after enquiring at the Embassy about possible restrictions related to the cholera epidemic in Afghanistan, went off to a rather seamy dive for lunch. An amusing Turk joined us, probably to exploit his knowledge of English, and introduced us to a culinary delicacy, sheeps testicles. We agreed they were excellent, then enjoyed his inability to reply to our tongue-in-cheek request to know 'what they were'.

Next we headed north towards the Caspian sea. The more direct route to Afghanistan lies across the desert to the south, but that road is reputed to be extremely hot and thick with the demonic drivers of whom we had already seen enough. However, the decision nearly led to our undoing.

We were by now a little edgy about the time we were taking to get through Iran, so we all sat down to look at the map one night and it seemed likely that we could take a short cut over a mountain pass and thus save an entire day. In single file we slowly progressed up the road as marked on the map. As we got higher and higher we crept in closer and closer to the wall as the drop on our near side became more and more precipitous. Then to our horror we rounded a corner and found an over-turned lorry. All its occupants, twenty to thirty people, had been thrown over the edge of the chasm. People were crying, the lorry completely blocked the road. This was the first time I saw the team go to work. John, Barney and I hurried up the road to the scene of devastation, totally unprepared for what we were to find underneath the lorry: the driver, completely crushed by the weight of his cab as it turned over on him. We learned from the people that he had tried to jump out as he lost control on the corner. But most of the other people were not seriously injured, though a few required patching up, and the girls set to with a will and managed to cope with all the problems. Then we had the unenviable job of trying to turn all our cars round on the very narrow road, with tyres inches from the edge of an enormous drop. Taking a few of the passengers with us, we travelled back down the pass again, the day we had hoped to gain, having been lost.

On the Caspian we could relax. The sea was warm and we established ourselves on the beach for two days, doing little more strenuous than proving that this particular stretch of coast line is totally devoid of fish, before turning inland again and finding ourselves on the worst stretch of road we were to encounter. For 400 miles, in temperatures around the 100 degree mark, we battled our way over sand and gravel, over rocks and along cart tracks. A cloud of dust was the only indication of the car ahead and overtaking presented a very disagreeable problem. Then, just a mile short of reaching tarmacadam, an explosion drew us rapidly to a halt. This was the only major puncture of the entire journey. A sharp boulder had ripped a piece from the side of a tyre. We were thankful that nothing more drastic had occurred.

We pushed on fast for the Afghanistan frontier, and the following day found ourselves in the Afghan town of Herat, ablaze with colour and good humour, and we found it delightful. Horse carts filled the streets, bedecked with flowers. Fierce Afghan faces broke into wide grins. Everything was cheap, everything was fascinating. The girls were soon trying on coats and capes made from mink and mountain leopard, fox and bear, for this is a country that abounds in wild life.

Afghanistan is similar to Nepal in that it is a kingdom until quite recently remote from the rest of the world. From the jungles and swamps in the south the land climbs away northwards through cruel desert to the fierce mountains of the Hindu Kush and the Russian border. The population is mostly nomadic, and a decade ago there were no roads at all. Only camel tracks crossed desert and mountain alike. Today a wide metalled surface, built by Russian and American aid programmes, runs from Iran to Pakistan, linking up with further roads virtually carved out of the mountains of the Hindu Kush.

Road-building in Afghanistan presents many problems, not least of these being the 'flash storm'. A heavy fall of rain in the mountains can transform a dry riverbed into a roaring torrent and across the barren desert a wall of water pours southwards carrying rocks as large as houses and destroying all in its path. A German engineer in the mid-twenties, who had designed many great bridges in Europe, built over twenty bridges in Afghanistan. All were destroyed by these terrible storms and failure drove him to suicide. A few pillars still remain as his epitaph.

Bridges today are flanked by great culverts which force the tidal wave to spread sideways, thus protecting the structure of the bridge itself. For drivers, these culverts can be very disconcerting as they produce the same effect as a Big-Dipper.

Between Herat and Kandahar lies pitiless desert. The sun blazes down out of cloudless skies, dust storms haze the horizon, life is stilled. In the middle of this inhospitable area we found a Mercedes bus which had broken down thirty-six hours before. The driver, a Scot, and his collection of rather scruffy hippy passengers were being held to ransom by an Afghani lorry driver who was demanding 100 American dollars to take them in tow.

They had no suitable tools with which to repair their vehicle: a clear example of bad preparation, we thought. But Peter was soon busy and he located the cause of all the trouble — a valve embedded in a piston head. After four hours of very hot work we immobilised the particular cylinder and cut off its diesel fuel supply, enabling the vehicle to limp on its way towards the inevitable destination — Kathmandu. John and Barney meanwhile had taken the opportunity to practice their rock-climbing on an inhospitable chunk of Afghani granite.

Kabul, city of bloodshed and terror, of beauty and hideous squalor, is magnificently situated at 7000 feet, surrounded by the snow-capped foothills of the Hindu Kush. If Genghis Khan had reappeared at the head of five thousand horsemen no-one would have been the least surprised. The British Embassy lies just outside the city in what must be one of the most delightful settings of any Residency in the world. Yet it is perhaps a tribute to our national stoicism that Britain has continued to maintain diplomatic relations with this amazing country, for on two separate occasions the entire Embassy staff has been murdered here.

We spent two days in Kabul and met up with Jo and Norman Harris, owners of Asian Greyhound tours. Norman is an Australian who had been running buses from the U.K. to Kathmandu for ten years when we met him. His tours are well organised and cheap, and he probably holds the record for overlanding. Certainly there is little he does not know about it.

From there we headed for Pakistan, and arrived at the frontier only to find that we were too late to cross the Kyber Pass, since this is not permitted after dusk. The whole area is controlled by tribal bands who ignore the authority of the Pakistani Government and have the unfortunate habit of shooting indiscriminately at vehicles and their occupants. We spent a nervous night in the garden of the customs post with two trigger-happy armed guards as escort.

The Kyber is disappointing, remarkable only for its memories of a calamitous defeat. The weather became hotter, unpleasantly so, and we resorted to wet towels to keep ourselves human. Salt tablets produced nausea and tempers became more frayed. Our object became only to get out of the searing heat.

After crossing the border into India we turned due north and drove up the mountain road towards the miraculous cool of Simla, where we spent a night in the Tibetan refugee camp perched high above the town.

The evening was made for us when we all crowded into Major Sweeney's upstairs room, Tibetans and our team, and listened to his tape recording of a prayer written by the

Dalai Lama. I found myself watching the faces of the little children, who are completely captivating, and catching their confidence that somehow, someday, they would return to the country which was their own. Stateless, in an alien environment, often unable to obtain work, these Tibetans maintain a serenity, a sense of humour and a joy in living that we all found deeply impressive.

The following morning before we left, as the sun rose above the ice-faces of the Hindu Kush, we were roused by the children's excited voices and got up to play with them on their swings in the courtyard outside the house.

In Delhi members of the High Commission staff did everything possible to make us feel at home. We were able at last to relax, and even to celebrate when John and Sheena decided to announce their engagement. Although this development was no surprise to the rest of us, we felt that the fact that their relationship had been forged over 6000 extremely difficult miles boded very well for their future.

The final stretch from Delhi to Raxaul on the Nepal border proved the most difficult of all. With the temperature over 100 degrees we battled our way east through dirt and dust, oxcarts and bicycles. A brief visit to the Taj Mahal was marred by the oppressive heat, and, crossing our final border at Birgung, we stopped for petrol in a record temperature of 120 degrees F. We made a headlong dash for the hills.

The road to Kathmandu was the first road to be built in Nepal, apart from those in the capital, and it was completed in 1963 with Indian aid. For seventy-eight miles it climbs up into the mountains, rising to 8000 feet, and this spectacular airy driving requires considerable concentration, strong wrists and a cool head.

At a height of 7500 feet, cool at last, we spent the night at Daman where an enterprising Nepali has built a miniature post-office tower. Only forty feet high and non-revolving, it permits one of the most spectacular views of the Grand Himal in the whole of Nepal. At five we were awake to watch the sun rise, lighting first Annapurna and Dhaulagiri in the west, then Langtang and Gauri Shankar, Lhotse, Everest and finally shining upon Makalu in the east.

The final stretch was upon us. We stopped for two hours just outside the city to clean up. The cars were washed and polished; and local Nepalis gazed in wonder at Penny doing the ironing on a bridge. Ties and suits, cotton dresses and make-up appeared from suitcases, and at 4.30 p.m. on May 28th 1969 we drove in through the gates of the British Embassy in a blinding rainstorm.

CHAPTER VII

Kathmandu

On the steps of the Embassy to greet us were the Ambassador, Arthur Kellas, and the Information Secretary, Dudley Spain. Arthur was an imposing figure with long sideboards and a bristling moustache; Dudley rather rotund and immediately identifiable as ex-army. He was, I think, a trifle taken aback to find us all dressed as if we had just walked out of a London hotel rather than travelled 7000 miles in a truck! And indeed at the time several members of the team probably thought the effort at smartness quite unnecessary. But it made a deep impression on the Ambassador and his staff, and I think we were justified in going to a lot of trouble to do just that.

The Ambassador's wife was away at the time and he was living in what looked like a typically English country house. Perhaps he was lonely, but it was also generosity that made him invite Penny and me to stay with him. We stayed for nearly seven weeks, and whenever I expressed misgivings about imposing so long on his hospitality, he would insist that he enjoyed having us and that it did not matter for how long. Penny indeed soon found herself involved with his social life, helping to arrange some of his many dinners and to entertain his guests.

It was at this time that I realized what a difficult job an Ambassador has. He has to maintain contact with all his own staff, while all the time extending and consolidating his contacts with the country in which he lives. Arthur Kellas did this with tremendous patience and considerable enthusiasm and good humour. I particularly remember his dry comment at a party to which we were invited with him by the American Ambassadress, to celebrate the tenth anniversary of the U.S. Embassy in Kathmandu: he didn't really understand, he said, why the Americans were celebrating their tenth anniversary! Why, only one year previously, he had not bothered to arrange a celebration of the one hundred and fiftieth anniversary of British connection with the country! We learned a lot from him and there is no doubt whatsoever that our Trust would not have survived without his able and ready assistance.

Dudley Spain was a great figure in Kathmandu, a bachelor, a great socializer and a very good diplomat. He opened doors for us, supplied the information we required, and was constantly arranging little gatherings of people that he thought we should meet.

To ease the frustrations of the waiting time, we dealt with official formalities such as medical registration, visited local hospitals and made short journeys into the surrounding country. Slowly our knowledge of the country and its people, its legend and history, its foundations and future aims, grew. We also took Nepali lessons.

There are many tribes in Nepal and they all have their own language. The common language is Nepali which basically stems from Sanskrit, and is used by almost everybody in the country. It is a very simple language to learn although I must confess that I never became very fluent myself — Penny, however, with her constant contact with servants and with her *ayah,* became virtually fluent within a year or so. To be able to carry on a reasonable conversation should take the average person only three or four months. Our chosen teacher was small and dapper. He was probably setting out to teach us perfect Nepali — as we would say in this country, the Queen's English — but his aim was too high, perhaps, and we were coming to the point when we would no doubt be able to speak very correctly to the Royal family, but not to converse with the ordinary people of the country, with whom after all we were going to have most of our dealings!

Nepal is a kingdom of eleven million inhabitants, 500 miles long and on the average 100 miles from north to south. To the north lies the greatest mountain chain in the world, bordering on Tibet (China): to the west lies Kumaon, and to the east, Sikkim. The southern border abuts on the dusty plains of India, the states of Uttar Pradesh and Bihar.

To the Westerner, perhaps, the name Nepal brings to mind pictures of Everest and Kanchanjunga, of snow and icy wastes — and no doubt of the world's bravest fighting men, the Gurkhas. But it is in fact a land of enormous scenic variety, and great cultural contrasts. It includes infinite beauty, extreme wealth and bitter poverty. From the great mountains in the north the land falls away in a series of steps until it flattens out into a thick jungle belt and then into the torrid areas of the plains. This lower belt is thirty to forty miles in depth, collectively known as the Terai, and it contains approximately half the population.

Until 1950 Nepal was virtually unknown to the outside world, few foreigners ever having crossed its borders. The country was ruled by the Rana regime, under a system essentially feudal. But in 1950 a great change occurred. Power was assumed by the King, who expressed his eventual intention of turning the country into a modern democracy. Twenty-five years later the king is still the overall governor of the country and all final decisions are made by him and him alone; but the modernisation of the country has undoubtedly gone ahead, the power of the feudal lords been weakened and the biggest discrepancies between rich and poor at least diminished. Many of the old Rana palaces have disappeared. Few families now have the enormous numbers of servants that were possible under the Ranas, who were divided into three classes, each of which was allowed a specific number of wives and concubines and a specific number of servants. This meant that there was a small number of very rich families, whilst the majority were very poor indeed. The revolution of 1950 was to begin to change the whole framework of that society, and the King's great achievement was to recognise his country's potential situation in a modern world, placed as it is between Tibet (China) and India, between Communism and Capitalism. India and China now compete to provide aid, and thus to influence Nepal's development. Nepalese policy is to accept aid equally from both sides and yet remain, as far as possible, apart from the tensions of the mightier nations. I often think of Nepal's future as that of a little Switzerland of the East: and like that of Switzerland, its economy is deeply dependent on tourism and agriculture, with only minor industry. Without tourism, indeed, Nepal could never develop and would always have to rely on outside aid.

With the coming of Western money and influence, the people in recent years have tended to drift down from the mountains into the towns and on to the plains. Many Gurkha soldiers for instance, who have served with the Indian or the British Army, return home to their hill towns only to become bored and dissatisfied with rural life, and migrate again to the larger areas of commerce and industry.

The principal magnet of course is Kathmandu, though it is only one of three cities in the Kathmandu Valley, which lies in the lower foothills of Nepal at a height of just over 4000 feet. Forty miles long and fifteen miles wide, the valley is reputed once to have been a lake, until a mythical giant (Manjushree) sliced away a gorge in the southern mountains so that the water ran away and revealed the lush and fertile soil we see today, drained by the Bagmati river.

Kathmandu, like its neighbouring cities of Patan and Bhadgaon, once had its own king and was independently governed. Then in 1767, out of the hills from Gorkha came Prithivi Narayan Shah, at the head of a powerful army. He laid siege to the town of Kirtipur, but met with such resistance that when the city finally fell, he cut off the noses and lips of all the inhabitants except the children and certain musicians, in reprisal for his own losses. Then he went off to attack the three major cities, which he defeated one by one, finally uniting the whole of Nepal under his own leadership.

The inhabitants of the Kathmandu Valley are predominantly Newar, traditionally the craftsmen of Nepal: the architects — whose finest works perhaps are the magnificent temples in Patan —, wood carvers, poets and musicians responsible for most of the art found in the valley today. But few craftsmen still practise their arts, many of which are lost for ever.

It is difficult to describe Kathmandu as it is today. The old city stands aloof from the new: dirty rambling streets form the Bazaar, opening out into squares where pagoda-style temples rear into the sky, decorated with erotic sculptures, which seemed to me at first sight hideous, though when I looked more closely I saw that they were superbly modelled in wood, brass, silver and gold. The ugliest of all Buddhas commands one such square; in lurid colours he dominates and appeals. Gigantic temples, Buddhist and Hindu, tower over scampering monkeys in their grounds.

Great palaces, relics of the Rana Regime, are now hotels and Embassies — the largest of all is Singha Durbar, the seat of Government. Once the largest private residence in the world, with 2000 rooms, it now provides space for 10,000 Civil Servants. A tangle of rooms forms a maze without exit — you have the feeling there that, even if by any chance you find the correct department, your prospect of ever seeing daylight again is purely a matter of chance.

The new city boasts modern hotels, an airport, wide, well-lit streets, modern offices and comfortable private houses: the contrast is incongruous, but characteristic of the suddenness with which development has come.

Within five or ten yards of the modern city you can find the most squalid conditions of the old city itself, the old Bazaar. It has been described as the town sitting on the biggest sewer in the world: you only have to go down the back streets to see the pathways being used as toilets by the children, and people throwing their refuse out of the windows. In some of the buildings there are great holes down the middle where, from whatever floor they are living on, the residents simply throw all their refuse into an enormous pit, and every year or so it is collected. The consequent indescribable smell is somehow just part of Kathmandu.

You walk down the main street of the Bazaar and you see children naked, passing motions right next to a fruit stall. You see the cows, even great big black bulls, wandering down the street helping themselves to vegetables. Cowpats and urine litter the footways. And, mixing shoulder to shoulder with the scruffy and the dirty, you see the American tourists waving their cameras, their sunglasses firmly clasped round their faces, and the hippies, their eyes glazed by marijuana — which is freely available in Kathmandu. There are scruffy hippies, and clean hippies, hippies of all races, German, American, Swedish, Norwegian, British and French.

Everyone comes to Kathmandu. The shops remarkably enough, are nearly always run by Indians. The restaurants range from the very good, which are very expensive, down to some Tibetan restaurants where you can get a very adequate meal for ten or fifteen pence.

At the airport, the taxi drivers try to extort whatever they can for the trip into the city. They can always pick out the person who's not going to be surprised when he's told that it will cost him twenty-five rupees, though the real figure is about eight or ten rupees. Yet nobody makes any effort to put a stop to the racket.

From Kathmandu you can fly all over the country. But it's difficult to get a ticket. And when you get to the airport, you may wait for a flight which doesn't exist, or the 'plane's not there purely because the monsoon rains have come. You get off two hours late — again this is part of Kathmandu. Very few people complain — they just accept it.

Air traffic has built up immensely over the last few years, so the airport is being enlarged to accommodate the larger jets. Caravelles landing with parachutes provided much enjoyment for the local populace, and not so long ago almost everyone in Kathmandu turned out to watch the first Boeing arrive, carrying the German President. After a trial run on the day before the State Visit, the pilot decided that he could make it; but not everyone was quite so confident and many decided to come along and watch the fun. The pilot did make it with a few feet to spare and it is rumoured that His Majesty the King immediately decorated both the President and the pilot for their bravery. To take off again proved even more difficult and most of the seats had to be removed to obtain the lift required to raise the huge jet from the runway.

Nepal is the only Hindu Kingdom in the world, but the country has a large Buddhist minority — the Buddha's birthplace is in fact at Lumbini in Western Nepal — and it is not at all uncommon to find Hindus and Buddhists worshipping in the same temples. Religious tolerance is characteristic of Nepal, and extends not only to the Buddhists but to the Muslims and other smaller religious groups.

The present King's system of government might be described as a party-less democracy, and it rests on the *Panchayat* system. The people of each village *(Gaon)* elect a *Panchayat,* or council, which in turn elects members to the District *Panchayat,* Zonal *Panchayat,* and finally to the National *Panchayat,* which is an Assembly composed of representatives of the Zonal *Panchayats* together with nominated specialists in certain fields, such as health, education, communication or the law. The development of communications, both within the country and with the outside world, has been one of the main preoccupations of the King's regime, for it is the key to the future fate of this geographically isolated country.

Flying in Nepal is not an easy undertaking at the best of times, though the record for disasters is probably one of the best in the world. Downdraughts from the mountains quickly transform a cloudless sky into dense mist and rain, yet with unerring accuracy the pilots pick their way through the mountains and drop down on to one of the many small grass landing-strips.

The *Raj Path* by which we entered Kathmandu, however, remains the only road leading south to India, and all supplies either come up this road or by the cable railway that threads its aerial way through the lower hills. Two years ago a new trade route was opened to the north-east, built by the Chinese, to join Kathmandu with the ancient capital of Tibet, Lhasa, and one further mountain road runs due north to Trisuli, where hydro-electric power is produced to supply the valley.

This road, carved out of the hillside, takes one past Kakani where the British Resident's summer home still stands high above the valley. It is now used for weekend release from Kathmandu. It is said once to have housed a huge mirror which was used to signal down to Kathmandu when further supplies of whisky were required! The view from here is breathtaking: to the north lies the Grand Himal, to the south the whole panorama of the ancient cities of the Kathmandu valley, often lying deep in dust and cloud in the early summer mornings.

During the monsoon, from early June until October, Kathmandu is humid and wet. From October to February the sun shines during the day, and the nights are cold. Then in the pre-monsoon period, the temperature gradually rises with the dust and the tourists crowd in. There are air flights to Everest, daily temple tours, elephant rides in tiger country — time to say hello and goodbye. The onset of the monsoon in June drives dust and tourists away and the cycle is completed.

It was now June, the monsoon was upon us, but the monotony of waiting for the formalisation of our contract was soon to be broken. John and Sheena were to be married. And if getting married in England involves much preparation, marriage in Kathmandu requires not only preparation but also a great deal of improvisation which in turn gave us a great deal of fun and made us many friends. Barney was best man, Gill bridesmaid and I was asked to give the bride away. Father Moran from St Xavier's School was to take the service. He was a small grey-haired figure, a bustling character with a good sense of humour and a great love of people, who had lived in Kathmandu for over twenty years. His school took children from all over the country and gave them an excellent education.

Boris Lisanovitch, a White Russian now a naturalised Englishman, renowned in Nepal for his sense of humour and readiness to do anything for anyone, made the cake and arranged the catering. The Embassy gardens were stripped of flowers. John and Sheena respectively embarked on the none-too-easy task of having a new suit and a wedding dress made; urgent cables flew backwards and forwards to England; invitations were printed, presents arrived. Barney added the spark of genius by hiring the only elephant in Kathmandu from the local zoo. And the morning of June 20th dawned a trifle indistinctly for all those who had attended John's stag party.

The service was held in the tiny chapel of St Xavier's, and after the ceremony John and Sheena mounted the elephant and a little precariously set off. Fortunately the rain held off until they were well on their way, and a landrover hovered close by to take them back to the Embassy for the reception. Speeches were made, the cake cut with a ceremonial *kukri,* and the couple departed in a shower of rice for their honeymoon in Pokhara.

We had had enough of Kathmandu, but still we were compelled to wait. Barney and Gill jumped the gun and went off to Biratnagar to find us somewhere to live. Peter set out for the squalor of Calcutta to make certain that our supplies had arrived; and then eventually on July 7th our contract was signed, initially for five years. The basic terms of the contract were that we were to be directly attached to the Directorate of Health Services and were to work in Kosi Zone in Eastern Nepal under the Zonal Health Officer — our base Biratnagar.

We took final leave of the Embassy and left Kathmandu just as we had entered, in blinding rain.

CHAPTER VIII

The British Connection

We were by now very much aware that Britain had a very special relationship with Nepal. This had an inauspicious beginning just over 150 years ago, when British troops were fighting the Nepalese. A dispute had arisen over whether certain areas on the southern border were in Indian or Nepalese territory.

Many fierce battles raged in the Terai and in the foothills of the Himalayas, over some of the most difficult terrain in the world. But the Gurkhas were fighting on their home ground and the British troops, under General Gillespie, were hurled back after bitter hand-to-hand fighting. Apart from the difficult terrain, the troops had to deal with fierce mosquito attacks which caused considerable casualties from malaria.

The arrival of General Octerlony proved the turning point of the war. A brilliant strategist, he skilfully attacked the Malaon fortress forcing the Nepalese General Amar Singh Thapa to surrender. By early 1816 British troops were in sight of Kathmandu, and to save further bloodshed a peace treaty was signed on March 4th 1816. By this treaty a large proportion of territory was taken over by the British, including parts of the Terai, Sikkim and Kumaon.

Deeds of bravery were celebrated on both sides and both commanders showed great chivalry to their enemies: General Octerlony described the Gurkhas as the bravest soldiers in the world.

Following the signing of the Treaty of Sagauli a British Resident was appointed to Kathmandu.

For thirty years after this war Nepal continued to suffer a period of great political unrest. There were repeated intrigues and assassinations, plots and poisonings. Then in 1845, after terrible bloodshed, Jung Bahadur Rana emerged as a national leader. He approved the British presence and did everything to foster friendship, offering Gurkha troops to fight in the Imperial army. He came to England in 1850, was received by Queen Victoria, and took the opportunity to study British laws and methods of administration. On his return to Nepal he devoted his energy to reforms, many of them on British models, with the result that British influence survives in the country to this day.

After a further period of unrest, in 1901 Chandra Shamsher became the country's leader. Well acquainted with England and its customs, it was he who was responsible for offering the entire Nepalese army to the British in the Great War of 1914 — an act of generosity possibly unique in international relations. After the war, in 1923, the treaty of 1816 was rescinded, Nepal recognised as an independent state, and a Nepalese Embassy was established in London. The Second World War saw the Gurkhas in action again, against the Germans in Europe and North Africa, and against the Japanese in Burma. Their courage and ferocity became a legend (thirteen men were decorated with the Victoria Cross for bravery beyond the call of duty in the years 1914-1945). The mere mention of the Gurkhas was said to have spread fear in enemy ranks.

In 1947, when independence was established in India, the Gurkha Brigade was divided — only three battalions remained under British control, the rest forming part of the Indian Army. They have continued to fight for Britain in Malaya, in Borneo and in Korea, always maintaining their record for unswerving loyalty.

Today, however, with the run-down in our overseas forces, few recruits are chosen each year, and the Gurkha Brigade may soon cease to exist. But there are still two recruiting bases, one at Dharan, north of Biratnagar, in the east, and the other in Paklihawa in the west. Dharan has been described as one of the most beautiful army bases in the world, situated on the edge of the jungle at a height of 1200 feet, overlooking miles of foothills. At both these bases, in addition to military training, courses are provided in agriculture, carpentry and bricklaying; and in Dharan a medical course has been added to the curriculum.

Further afield in Giri, just east of Kathmandu, and at Lumle, west of Pokhara, agricultural centres are being established which will provide ex-soldiers with training in improved methods of pest control, cultivation and animal breeding.

Indeed, one is frequently reminded in Nepal of the British connection. The Ambassador's residence reminds one of an English country house: the garden, laid out by Sir Christopher Summerhayes, is one of the finest in Kathmandu. On H.M. the Queen's Birthday seven hundred people pack the lawn, the Nepalese army band plays from the balcony and pipers provide a sort of cabaret. The Royal tent stands in the corner, liquor flows, Russians rub shoulders with Americans, Chinese with Israelis, the lawn is trampled and the driveway pitted by car wheels. Small as our Embassy is in comparison with others, it has a special, intimate status as though one hundred and fifty years of attachment has almost removed the brand of 'foreigner.' British assistance has helped found the All-Nepali broadcasting system, set up the local manufacture of pharmaceuticals, and will lead soon to the building of the first English-type Public School.

A quarter of a mile from the Embassy compound is the British Council, which has an excellent library, organises films and plays, recitals and exhibitions, and administers British volunteer services, such as the V.S.O. which provides occasional young people as nurses and teachers. Films are very popular, for the desire for knowledge is acute and the means for satisfying the hunger are few. Nepalese filmgoers are thus not always discriminating, and I well remember an evening when two reels of a Hitchcock thriller were followed by a final reel of the Marx Brothers, and the audience barely seemed to notice.

Goal, the film made about the 1966 football World Cup, was especially popular, and many people saw it through four or five times, for Nepalis love sport. A committee has now been established for the promotion of sport, headed by His late Majesty King Mahendra's son-in-law, Gyanendra. Football, hockey, cricket and table tennis head the list of popular games, and just outside the airport stands one of the most incredible golf courses I have ever seen. Once eighteen holes, now cut down by the runway to nine, it provides every hazard known to golf. Apparently innocuous fairways conceal hidden gorges sixty feet deep, a short drive finds one playing out of sticky mud or twelve-foot-high sweet-corn. The membership list includes Ambassadors and Generals, Princes and Maharajas. An open competition is held annually and matches are played against Dharan (the only other course in Nepal), and Dewars from India.

Tourist expansion however is now bringing other foreigners to Nepal. The industry not only means desperately required foreign currency but also a corresponding increase in demand for better accommodation and internal methods of communications and dramatic increases in land prices, food prices and labour costs. People flock down from the hills to work in the new hotels and the many service industries which spring up around tourism. They earn more money than they ever have before; but, in the towns at least, their money will buy them less, and like so many other developing countries, Nepal now has before it the ugly prospect of a growing urban working class vulnerable first to the consequences of local inflation, and even eventually to unemployment should an international slump at any time reduce the flow of visitors.

Nepal's future is now inextricably bound up with the fate of the world beyond the mountains.

CHAPTER IX

We Settle In

Biratnagar, the largest town outside the Kathmandu valley, has 100,000 inhabitants, and a catchment area of double that population. It lies in the Terai, three miles from the Indian border at Jogbani, with which it is connected by a British Gurkha-built road running from Jogbani to Dharan, thirty miles due north at the base of the foothills. As the seat of Government for Kosi Zone, Biratnagar controls a population of 800,000 people, of which approximately half live in the hills and half in the two Terai districts of Morang and Sunsari.

Industries include jute, which is exported all over the world, a sugar mill, stainless steel and textile plants, brick kilns and button and cigarette factories.

As we drove out of the airport into the dusty plains I was immediately struck by the heat and the humidity, the smell of jute rotting by the side of the road, and by the difference in the people, because many of them are of Indian origin. The bustle is there: the squalor outside the town itself, and then within the city little grubby houses thatched with banana leaves intermingle with the concrete of the new generation of two- or three-storey buildings, the shops on the ground floor overflowing on to the pavements with their silks and saris, sugar and rice. Cows still roam the streets, and buffalo as well, and the drainage system leaves much to be imagined.

We missed the greenery of the lush fertile Kathmandu valley — we had come down to the brown heat of the plain. Jute, rice and sugar grew all around us, but somehow it was a grey barren earth compared with what we had left.

Gill and Barney had found us a house, built to Western specifications only a year ago, but never inhabited. It lay in fairly open country on the south side of the town, 150 yards from the main road, so once a contract was drawn up and signed we had the satisfaction of at least having a roof over our heads. It was named Kafle Niwas.

Peter had also been successful in Calcutta, squeezing our supplies through the Customs department and the clearing agents. He had in fact performed something approaching a miracle. It is accepted in Nepal that fifteen to twenty per-cent of every consignment will be lost in transit through India. Goods are taken from boxes and replaced by bricks, bottles of whisky emptied by the simple expedient of putting a syringe through the cork and syphoning out the contents; milk powder is extracted from bags through bamboo shoots; cars are stripped of wing mirrors, batteries and even wheels. A battalion of Gurkhas would find it difficult to outwit the ingenuity of the Indian thieves. Yet thanks to Peter, we were to lose virtually nothing.

Settling in was a nightmare, and without the help of the Officers and men from the British Army recruiting centre at Dharan, we might have starved, or even drowned in our own garden. For a month chaos reigned. The house leaked like a sieve. We had a limited water supply, food was difficult to obtain, mainly because we did not know where to buy it — we learnt later that we should have employed a Nepali cook at once, who would have known how to forage for food. Cooking was done in rotation by the girls; and cooking for eleven on two primus stoves is hardship itself.

Slowly things were put into shape. The painting was finished and furniture was purchased locally. The garden was drained and, luxury of luxuries, a mains water supply installed. Plumbers in Nepal are at a premium, good plumbers very rare indeed, and a simple repair of a leaking pipe can result in a flood if you turn your back for an instant.

The arrival of three lorries from Calcutta with our supplies and personal luggage gave us more work, and also a welcome change of diet from soup and rather musty bread. But it was only with the arival of an ex-Gurkha cook from Darjeeling, and another ex-Gurkha bearer, that we were able to relax. Our cook was named Dhan Bahadur, but known as Baje (Grandfather) by the rest of the staff. In the past he had been a field-cook in the army, and in response to a letter sent to him in Darjeeling he had arrived on our doorstep and set to work without even discussing the question of his pay. This inscrutable man was the ruler of the Household and he astonished us in his first week by producing roast pork with superb crackling cooked in a saucepan on a single paraffin stove. As time went by our visitors were to increase, not only from Dharan but also from Kathmandu and from the scattered villages where our friends in the American Peace Corps were working. Yet at a moment's notice Baje would provide the extra food required, as if he had already known that an increase in numbers was likely.

And following him, came more staff, and a consequent transformation in our lives. Pemba Lama, a Sherpa, also from Darjeeling started as a sweeper at the princely sum of one pound a week with which he kept his wife, himself and their three children. His great ability to put his hand to anything soon achieved his promotion to bearer. Our gardener (Mali) was an ex-Gurkha Sergeant who had come to us when his home and all his land had been swept away by floods in the hills. An enormous man, he was highly recommended by the Brigadier from Dharan. How lucky we were! With a *kukri* always slung at his waist he presented an imposing figure and incidentally acted as a considerable deterrent to unwanted visitors. Somlal, our *dhobi* (laundryman), came to us very early on and never failed us. In three years he was absent only on four occasions, and on each of these he sent his brother to do his work. Mountains of washing went through his hands and even in the monsoon he managed to keep the supply running.

We were unaccustomed to the country, so we had found ourselves with paint brush in hand, or repairing pipes. But this is absolutely unheard of in Nepal. If you want to cut a patch of lawn, you don't do it yourself, you employ somebody to do it because it's a menial task. This was one of the first things the Nepalese commented on, and we saw their point of view and started to employ other people rather than try to be our own handymen.

The house was still not big enough for all of us, however, so John and Sheena moved into another house half a mile away, and Di and Vint into an empty flat in the hospital grounds.

At last we were ready to assume our proper roles of doctors and nurses. Our hospital work was about to begin.

Biratnagar had one hospital of forty beds conveniently divided between males upstairs and females down, with a small isolation unit apart from the main building. Four Nepali doctors were directly attached to the hospital, and a local practitioner supplied a limited Pathology service.

Most of the work by far was done in the Out-Patients department, in a building hopelessly inadequate to cope with the daily attendances. It was terribly small and was coping with a vast influx of people every day, so it was very difficult to organise. Teeming masses poured through that door — people with T.B., children with dysentery, skin diseases, leprosy, fractures, people who had fallen out of trees, anything you can think of came through that door every morning and doctors had to cope with case after case, only really finding three or four minutes for each one. Often the strongest would fight to get in first, and the staff would have to take time off to try to get some sort of queue organised again.

There is no doubt that initially we were too ambitious about our task, and a little hasty in our judgments. Eastern thinking is often at variance with our own, and the whole pace of life is slower and more reflective.

The aim of the Trust was quite clear and accepted by His Majesty's Government, namely to improve medical facilities wherever and whenever possible, only undertaking new projects which, in the fullness of time, would become an integral part of the Nepalese health structure totally staffed by Nepalis. But we tended to rush in with our ideas for improvement and development, and it took us some time to realise the extent of our own insensitivity.

Reverse the situation and try to imagine a team of Nepalis arriving in Brighton and setting about the reorganisation of the Group Management Committee, unable to speak English and ignorant of British customs and local attitudes. It says a great deal for the Nepali staff in Biratnagar that virtually no attempt was made to curb our enthusiasm.

Looking back, I can now see how remarkable it was that the Zonal Health Officer, Dr Baidya, a man who is now Director of Health for the whole country, and the other senior doctors in the hospital, accepted us. We were all comparatively young. We moved in with a good deal of enthusiasm and a singular lack of knowledge of the country, and proceeded to break down walls and put in concrete sinks and goodness knows what else, all in a sort of flash of optimism, and in true Eastern fashion, they were able to sit by and watch. They very rarely made any comments, either favourable or unfavourable, and it wasn't really until we'd done a tremendous amount that we stopped to think that Dr Baidya had in fact designed this hospital, and seen it built, and now he was watching people from a country 7000 miles away calmly walk in and destroy a lot of what he'd done. When I got to know him later on, he admitted that it was often difficult to do this.

The Out-Patient theatre was our first line of advance. We redecorated it and equipped it with new instruments and dressings. Then we turned an empty room in the hospital into a five-bedded childrens' ward, which was desperately needed because the weekly Maternal and Child Health Clinic dealt with over 100 patients. A Pathology Laboratory was running within six weeks, through the combined efforts of Di and Vint. This was the first fully equipped Laboratory outside the Kathmandu valley and provided an essential medical service.

Gill reorganised the Operating Theatre, Rosemary the Midwifery Unit, and Prue took over the Childrens' Ward. John was doing surgery, Penny anaesthetics, Sheena was on the male ward and we all worked in Out-Patients, slowly learning the language. An efficient autoclaving system was established and urgently required drugs and equipment distributed to all departments.

We had received many adverse reports on Biratnagar during our sojourn in Kathmandu, mainly about the climate. Before the monsoon the weather is very hot and frequent dust storms blown by the easterly wind cover everything in a grey film. With the onset of the monsoon the temperature falls, the dust settles, but the humidity is strangely strength-sapping. Winter demands numerous blankets, heaters and warm clothing. October and November is the perfect time of the year: dew rises from the ground overnight and the mountains far off away to the north become ever more prominent as the snow line falls. But we found ourselves steadily acclimatised, and our second year was to find us donning sweaters when the temperature fell to 75 degrees F.

When we first arrived, the only other three Westerners living in the town were Hank, working for the United States AID programme in the field of malaria eradication, Bill, and Bill's wife Nancy, working for AID in agriculture. It was Bill who introduced us to the Honda motor cycle, which he drove with considerable verve and apparent impunity all over the Terai. Rivers and sand yielded equally to Bill and his machine, and only once was he defeated. Arriving at a particularly wide river during the height of the monsoon he dismounted to test the depth, which he did quite simply by stepping off the bank. As the water closed over his head he found himself thinking that even a Honda would have failed under those conditions.

Through Bill and Nancy we got to know many of the American Peace Corps Volunteers in our area, and soon they became regular visitors to our house. Peace Corps workers, like those of the British Voluntary Service Overseas, are sent to developing countries of the world to help in education and in agriculture. At a preliminary training course they are taught the language of the country and prepared for the difficulties which they are likely to encounter. They are expected to spend a minimum of one year living in a village, and to become an active part of the community in which they find themselves. It is quite remarkable that so many of these men and women are able to adapt themselves to the very difficult and lonely world into which they are projected, and I was very impressed by the standard of their work. This was particularly apparent in the field of agriculture, where they are able to introduce new methods of crop control and breeding and even in some cases entirely new crops.

Jack was someone we particularly liked. He was about twenty-three, and he worked in a school in Biratnagar so we saw a great deal of him. He loved the country, he loved the people but like all of us he found Eastern attitudes at times hard to come to terms with, though he was making continual efforts to adapt himself. Sometimes he grew a moustache, at others he chopped it off again. He changed, as his attitudes changed, sometimes depressed, sometimes enthusiastic. But above all he wanted to make sure that the examinations in his school were properly conducted, and when he discovered that many of the students had been cheating, he came to us in despair. In some schools this custom had been accepted; but Jack was having none of this and he made quite sure that the exams were held again and done correctly. He won out, and the students regarded him with considerable respect for what he had done.

He became so well integrated with his school that none of the discretion normally due to a foreigner was shown to him at the festival of Holi. This festival, usually held at the beginning of March, is one of the most important of the Hindu year and is characterised by the indiscriminate use of paint and coloured powder which is thrown, squirted and squeezed at almost anyone and anything. Only policemen are exempt and old clothes are the order of the day. No-one recognised Jack when he appeared in our drive covered from head to foot in paint. His hair was a delicate shade of blue and the rest of him resembled a rainbow. He had been waylaid by his fellow teachers and given the full treatment. It took him nearly two weeks to return to his normal colour. We joined in with abandon and found that Gentian Violet and Malachite green produced an excellent, if rather enduring, result.

Almost the very first patient in Biratnagar presented me with a dog, which we immediately christened Makalu. Of uncertain ancestory, he looked like a cross between a Basset hound and a Queen Anne chair. He was the first of a series of pets to join our household, which included Gill's Tibetan terrier, Seamus, a parrot (eaten whole by Makalu), a rabbit (which died of shock when faced with Seamus), and a cat.

CHAPTER X

A Working Day

Once everything had settled into a routine many of the complications and arguments of the early days could be avoided. Nearly everyone knew what the others were doing at least a week ahead, and it became possible to prevent situations in which someone required a car to go to the Hospital ten minutes before the main body of the team wanted to leave. In fact when no car was available matters became even simpler, as everyone made his or her own arrangements. Two motor cycles were bought, and three bicycles, which trebled the overall mobility of the team. Nurses going into the hospital at 7.30 a.m. would go on bicycles and others could follow in the car if it was available, or on the motor cycles: girls riding motor cycles caused something of a stir in the town and the Nepali nurses gazed in wide-eyed amazement.

We usually tried to start a Ward Round at 8.30 a.m., but all too often a multitude of small queries would make us late, much to the disgust of the nursing staff. Rounds would be conducted in much the same way as they would be in England, except that there was no division between medical and surgical cases, every doctor being expected to know about each case. We always tried to keep the cases of active tuberculosis segregated from the other patients, but this was often impossible, as a patient admitted with a fractured femur would frequently turn out to have tuberculosis as well.

Shortage of beds was always a problem, especially in the expanding Midwifery Unit, where, if there were no complications at delivery, mother and child were sent home after twenty-four hours to make way for the next arrival. On Wednesday of each week the routine was altered to cope with the Maternal and Child Health (M.C.H.) Clinic. Home visiting by the nurses encouraged mothers to bring their children to this clinic at regular intervals, so that their progress could be judged and treatment given when required. Smallpox and B.C.G. vaccinations were given and also Triple Vaccine, when available, to protect against diphtheria, whooping cough and tetanus. All medicines were supplied free of charge; and so also was milk for those in particular need. It was very encouraging to see the general standard of hygiene and health improving over the years, and the rise in attendance as more and more mothers became aware of the services offered. For many mothers this was a 'day out', and women in their very best saris would arrive with impeccably dressed children. Heavily tattooed Tharu girls would rub shoulders with Marawaris, Brahmins with Limbus and Chettris with Rais.

On operating days the physician would normally complete the round in the hospital whilst the anaesthetist and surgeon departed to theatre. Meanwhile, in the small Out-Patient Department, two doctors tried desperately to cope with a tide of humanity which started to pour through the doors at half past seven every morning.

We soon found ourselves in need of a secretary and were fortunate enough to obtain the services of an ex-Gurkha, Mr Dewan, who did a great deal of our typing and acted as Registration Clerk in the mornings, endeavouring to ensure that everyone ended up in the correct department.

We rarely had lunch before two o'clock and the nurses were often much later, so we tended to eat in relays, limiting ourselves to something simple such as soup, omelette and the occasional curry, which lightened the workload for our cook and bearer.

After lunch was the time for general administration: replying to correspondence, writing reports, checking the accounts, paying staff and a host of other matters that seemed never to end. Lemon tea brought a welcome respite, then the arrival of the postman, an interlude of excitement sometimes dampened by the thought that the round of letter-writing had to start again.

Showers and rum followed in the early evening, and by eight we were usually sitting down to the main meal of the day. Mealtimes were a good time for discussion, but often, after a long day, conversation palled and we retired to bed early.

CHAPTER XI

Into the Hills

Although we were based at Biratnagar, we did not feel that our responsibilities stopped at the edge of the plain. After all, it was to the hill country that we had been attracted in the first place, so within a few weeks of arrival Barney, who had more energy than anyone, set off for the hills to assess the conditions in Dankhutta in case part of the team should be required there at some time in the future. Although the monsoon was at its peak, which makes trekking extremely uncomfortable, he slipped and slithered his way north with his usual enthusiasm, doing daily battle with the tenacious leeches.

The trail leaves Dharan Bazar and climbs steeply upwards to the top of the Sanguri ridge at an altitude of 5000 feet, then dives down again at an even steeper angle to a tiny village nestling in the shadow of high cliffs in the angle formed by two rivers, which in the monsoon can become raging torrents.

From here the trail sidles along the river bank until it reaches the mighty Tamur river. Two hundred feet wide, this torrent rages along at twenty knots carrying all before it, but fortunately it is spanned by a suspension bridge built by the Gurkha Engineers almost thirty years ago. Everyone and everything crosses this bridge and sometimes a hurried retreat becomes necessary as a wide-eyed frightened cow gallops across from the other side. In the wind the bridge sways quite noticeably and one nervously quickens one's pace to reach the haven of the tea shops on the further side. Every village is well supplied with tea shops and the hot sticky tea is a marvellous restorer of energy on a weary journey.

After a rest the second ridge has to be tackled, winding its way up through tiny villages, until three hours later Dankhutta comes in sight.

Dankhutta is typical of many of the hill towns of Nepal, in that it is magnificently situated, perched on a saddle and surrounded by forested valleys, but difficult of access. You approach it up a winding hill which only a landrover could negotiate, and that with difficulty, for the road rises in long cobbled steps, a water pipe running down its side. As you go up thatched houses give way to more substantial ones, with wooden balconies overlooking the street, and flowers in window-boxes on the corners. There is a bustle of animals and people walking endlessly up and down in a never-ending stream.

Dankhutta itself runs for about a mile, threading through the bazaar to an open space of ground where the weekly market is held. This is a great occasion to which people from all the surrounding areas bring their wares: grapefruit and oranges, apples and vegetables and occasionally meat. Meat is difficult to come by, but due to the enthusiasm of the Peace Corps Volunteers and some of the local people, pigs are now being bred in the area. One Peace Corps Volunteer actually carried his pig in over the hills so that a new strain could be bred suitable for the hill country!

It is a town of about 6000 people, and I suppose its architecture could best be compared to that of an old Tudor town in England, well cared-for in parts, decrepit in others, its beauty in its higgledy-piggledy disorder.

The Government hospital is at the lower end of the town, rather drab behind cold grey walls. Lying in its own compound, it was dealing with sixty to seventy out-patients daily and had twelve beds for the more serious cases. The local Government officials were enthusiastic about the possibility of our sending a team to work there, and very soon Barney was discussing their difficulties.

It seemed in particular that the hospital was desperately short of drugs, especially antibiotics, and that the few medicines available in the shops in the town were prohibitively expensive. Within a few days of his return to us Barney was busy working out a scheme by which medicines could be supplied to the hill towns at a reasonable rate, and plans were being made to put the scheme into operation.

We felt that it would be a good idea to have a look at all the main health facilities in our zone, and as the monsoon was coming to an end (so we thought) it was decided that the other centres should be visited. I was to go; and Keith, a young Gurkha Officer in charge of the welfare of retired Gurkha soldiers, who had to make frequent treks into the hills to visit the soldiers' homes, was willing to accompany me. I was to be very grateful for his company, not least because he had a fluent command of Nepali.

On September 30th 1968 we left Dharan following the same route as Barney had done. As soon as we reached the base of the hills in and around the Bazar we were in a world of richness and colour. The drabness of the hot plain gave way to gay costumes, gold rings in the nose, colourful shawls and bright topis. Tibetan women came down from the high hills and, as you climbed up the steep road towards Dankhutta, the porters passing you on their way had smiling faces. There was a great casualness about the way of life, and yet terrific friendliness — nearly everybody would say something to you as you passed on the road, often very small talk, but kindly. Someone might say 'Where are you going?' and you would reply 'Up', or 'Down'. There is no offence taken at this brevity, for in Nepal a reply to the question 'What's the time?' might be simply: 'Late' — greeted with a sort of grin. Such exchanges are simply expressions of recognition — like 'Isn't the weather nice?' in England.

We soon learned to adjust to small things like this — such as the Nepali tendency to laugh at other people's predicaments. If you slipped over in the mud or fell into a stream, this was greeted by roars of applause and laughter which took us aback at first. And then, quite obviously, it was funny and, unless you'd been seriously injured — which didn't happen very often — you had a laugh with them; and when one of your porters slipped off a bridge, you just sat there and shook at him. These little things made the walks in the hills cheerful affairs.

The hill porters often suffered from tuberculosis, and yet they were fantastically fit men. One man I remember walking very slowly up behind us, sat down in the same tea shop, and when he put his basket off his shoulders on to the floor I looked at it and saw it to contain at least four four-and-a-half-gallon cans of kerosene and a good deal else, so I asked him if I could see if I could lift it. I could *just* get it off the floor. He was carrying this happily into the hills! Yet the men carrying these enormous weights never suffer from any neck trouble. I suppose they train themselves, because they exercise their neck the entire time. Most of the weight rests on the head, carried by a headband. And very rarely do you meet a gruff or grumpy porter.

We reached Dankhutta as night was falling. The weather had been hot and sticky and a light drizzle floated in a mist all around us. Then next morning as we travelled north from Dankhutta through the lovely village of Hile, the clouds became thicker and we moved like shadows in a silent land. Hile had sprung suddenly into existence in 1953 when the closure of the northern border forced many of the Bhotias to move south in search of trade. Almost entirely Buddhist, it is a happy colourful town liberally sprinkled with Tibetan rugs and carpets. The ridge from Hile to Terathum can offer one of the most magnificent views in Eastern Nepal, but our luck was out and we had difficulty in finding the path, let alone catching a glimpse of the Himal. Our porters looked grim and muttered that it was likely to get worse, and our sagging spirits sank still further.

In Terathum we found a busy Health Post manned by a

nurse and a Health Assistant. It was short of medicines but not of patients, so it was not very long before I was running a clinic dishing out my limited supplies to a never-ending stream of complainants. A splendid old woman who looked about one hundred and five but was probably not older than fifty produced an enormous marrow from her bag and insisted that I take it for my consultation.

Then, armed with further experience of local medical problems and my marrow, we headed out again for the village of Tembe, where I was to meet for the first time one of the most charming men I ever could wish to know — Honorary Lieutenant Kalu Sing Limbu, who had retired from the army ten years before after a long and distinguished career, returned to his village in the hills, and set himself to improve not only his home but the entire village.

I am quite certain that a bush-telegraph system operates in the hills of Nepal, for somehow or other people always seem to know when you are coming. Kalu greeted us at the door of his two-storeyed house, remarking quite casually that we must have lost our way as we should have been there some two hours earlier. How he could possibly have known this I do not understand for no one had passed us on the trail. But we were soon sitting, happily relaxed in his collapsible chairs — purchased in Singapore — and being liberally served with curry and rice beer. Kalu was in the middle of his daily 'Out-Patients Clinic'. Without any previous medical training he was taking excellent histories and distributing the required medicines with precision.

Kalu speaks English perfectly but prefers to speak in his native tongue in a slow and measured manner so that even I was able to gather the gist of the conversation. In his area were many ex-Gurkhas and he was able to give Keith an accurate description of all their requirements and difficulties. After our meal he took us on a tour of inspection of his village to show us the improvements he had made. A very lively school dominated the village and alongside he was building a small dispensary to be staffed by an ex-army medical orderly. Piped water ran between the houses and plans were afoot to build fish tanks, and a fence against wild animals. All this had been achieved by his enthusiasm which in turn had stimulated the villagers. Equipment and labour were provided free by the local people. I only wish that more soldiers returning to the hills would take Kalu as an example of what can be achieved.

That night we fell asleep to the sound of heavy rain and the barking of Kalu's four enormous mastiff dogs.

We were tempted to stay longer but days were slipping by and we had work to do. The mountains away to the north lay shrouded by thick cloud, imposing an air of impending doom all around us. We hurried on and just as we reached the village of Chainpur the sky split apart and the most torrential storm that I have ever seen, such as I never wish to see again, began. Thunder roared overhead and sheets of lightning lit up the sky. The rain came down in a solid wall and soon the main street of the village was two feet deep in mud-coloured water. Fortunately we were able to find shelter in a tiny house at the top of the main street which served as a pension-paying post for the Ghurkhas of the Indian Army.

Two rooms about eight feet square were to be our home for the next seventy-two hours. There was only one tiny window and the smoke from the fire clung around us and stung our eyes. The only way to obtain respite was to sit on the floor with the door wide open. We played cards — almost every game known to man including thirty games of Canasta. Our porters were sent out to scrounge for food, only to find that little was available and that the village had been cut off from the surrounding area by the rising floods. Down below us, a mile away, a river which two days before had contained only two feet of water was now a raging flood fifty feet across and twenty feet deep.

Only rice and lentils were available and this monotonous diet did little to improve our humour. So Keith and I decided to brave the rain and to go food-hunting on our own account, and we did manage to find a shop which sold biscuits and condensed milk. The shopkeeper was slightly taken aback when we devoured an entire packet of biscuits in front of him in about two minutes flat, washing them down with the rather thick milk.

A tremendous crack during our second night of continuous rain brought us from our sleeping bags with the agility of rabbits. The garden of the house next to us was slipping away before our eyes as the water undermined it, and after this incident we slept little, wondering whether we were to meet the same fate. At last a watery sun broke through the clouds and we got a glimpse of the great glacier face of Makalu, now very close to us in the north. Reports of landslides were ever more frequent and we realised that we would have to wait for several days for the rivers to fall before we could start on our homeward journey.

When we did get on our way again I was suddenly stricken with severe dysentery which failed to respond to any of the medicaments that I was carrying. I realised that I probably had amoebic dysentery which, although not serious, can prove very debilitating. My frequent trips to the bushes slowed our progress, and the havoc wrought by the storm impeded us still further.

All over the countryside landslides had forged giant paths of destruction carrying all before them. Houses and fields looked like battlefields, sections of the trail had disappeared completely and frequently we had to struggle across a moving morass of mud. The Arun river was our first major obstacle. Two hundred feet wide, it boiled along carrying trees and great boulders, even an occasional dead buffalo. There was no bridge so the only method of getting across was in a hollowed-out tree trunk poled by four enthusiastic hillmen. Our porters viewed the crossing with equanimity, which was even more surprising when I found out later that not one of them could swim a stroke. Sitting in six inches of water we cast off into the current, at first polling upstream in the back-eddies. Suddenly the current grasped us and with our oarsmen polling like demons we were swept out into the stream. Spray lashed our faces, tree trunks reared up at us from the water and the rapids drew startlingly closer. Just at the moment when all seemed lost the back-current gripped us and we staggered ashore four hundred yards downstream. Keith and I lit cigarettes with shaking fingers and the green hue slowly faded from our faces. .

When we reached Bhojpur we found a very enthusiastic doctor running a hospital of twenty-five beds. He welcomed us, showed us round and reiterated the old story: that his most desperate lack was of medicines. The Area Welfare Officer, an ex-Gurkha, not only provided us with excellent accommodation but also organised a display by local singers and dancers for us, and dawn was breaking before the gyrations had ceased.

Back across the Arun, we sighed with relief to be on the home stretch at last, and slowly wended our way back to Dharan. For my dysentery was much worse and if it had not been for Keith's perseverance I doubt if I could have made it back on my feet. The last mile took me almost two hours and gratefully I staggered into bed. I was to find later that I had lost over two stone in those three weeks, and only my tan belied my internal troubles.

We had fully confirmed Barney's conclusion that the best way to help in the hills would be to set up an organisation to supply medicines at a reasonable price, and it seemed logical that we should approach Indian companies for them. There are literally hundreds of pharmaceutical companies in India, but some of these are totally unreliable, and many are the accounts of antibiotic capsules being found to be full of nothing but sugar, so we had to select our suppliers carefully. We drew up a list of necessary preparations and tried to limit our sources to as few companies as possible. Armed with this list I set off on a round trip of India to see if I could get reduced terms on the items we required.

I arrived in Calcutta in a rainstorm, the streets were awash and the water was creeping up the steps of my Hotel. And floodwater in Calcutta is like no other water on earth. It is rumoured that in the great massacres that followed partition in 1947 countless human bodies were simply pushed into the sewage system but whether this is true or not there is no doubt that even when it is dry the drainage system cannot cope, and when it is wet one feels that the Ganges itself has invaded the city. The population is estimated at eight million but there could easily be double that number squeezed into the fragile shanties, and spilled out again on to the filthy streets. At night the town is covered in a pall of smoke from the hundreds of fires lit on the pavements where huddled forms grasp at the puny warmth. In the morning many will not get up, their corpses stiff in the position of the night before.

From Calcutta I flew south to Bombay where my friends David and Sally Symonds, who had entertained me on my first trip to Delhi, looked after me once more, and arranged for me to meet the Directors of various companies. Bombay still reflects a profound British influence, and I liked the open sea and wide streets in contrast to the crowded alleys of Calcutta. During the week that I spent there I visited eleven companies and in every case was received with great courtesy and encouragement. I was able to order most of the supplies we required, and in many cases the companies concerned were willing to donate some of their products. I also learned a great deal about the difficulties that beset the pharmaceutical industry in India, and especially how difficult it can be to introduce a new product from abroad. It seems that products passed by the Dunlop Committee in the United Kingdom must go through the complete process again in India, which may mean a lapse of two years before the drug is actually available on the Indian market.

I returned via Delhi and thence to Kathmandu where I had some matters to discuss with our Embassy and with the Health Department of the Government.

Back in Biratnagar Barney was building up his plans for distribution. In each area the local Panchayat officials were to choose a retailer to whom we would deliver the medicines as required. He would in turn estimate his requirements in collaboration with the local doctor or Health Officer. Since this was to be a non-profit-making scheme, it had to be organised in such a way that when the medicines reached the door of the retailer we would be able to tell him at what price the medicines could be sold in his shop, to cover the delivery costs and still enable him to make a modest profit himself. Ganga was our first retailer and of course he, as the guinea-pig, was in Dankhutta. Soon others were appointed and the system was established in five hill towns. The system when fully operational allowed the Health Officer in each town to utilise his small quantity of free medicines supplied by the Government for those desperately in need, and yet to prescribe preparations for others knowing that they were available at a reasonable price close at hand. Working with a capital of £1400 we were able to take stock at the end of two years and to show that we had made a loss of only £20, which says much for Barney's accuracy.

We now had one small operating theatre and a very eager Nepali surgeon in Biratnagar. The surgeon's name was Dr Bhattacharya. He had been trained in India and received his Fellowship in Edinburgh. Whilst working in Wales he had been given the name of 'Joe' since his forenames were held to be unpronounceable, and it took only a short acquaintance to find that this was indeed so, and to all of us he became 'Joe'.

Unlike many others who had found it difficult to readjust themselves on returning to Nepal, Joe relished the challenge and had succeeded in establishing two excellent district hospitals before coming to Biratnagar. He was able to cope with nearly all of the many dialects in the area, and had an astonishing flair for diagnosing patients on first appearance. He became a good friend and a great teacher. Before our arrival the Zonal Director, Dr Bharat Raj Baidya, and he had shared the medical and surgical cases, interchanging with each other when an anaesthetic was required.

The only anaesthetic possible at that time was 'Open-Ether', an ancient but very safe method. Then, thanks to the very good advice of Neville Ripley from Longworth's Scientific Instrument Company, we were supplied with an E.M.O. machine, which is the ideal instrument for giving anaesthetics under difficult conditions. This machine was to prove itself within a few months.

It seemed now that John Ward's services could best be used in Dankhutta, and after some fairly lengthy discussion it was decided that we should send a surgical team to establish an active operating centre there.

John and his wife Sheena, Vint and Di were to constitute the team. John as the surgeon, and his wife as Theatre Sister, were to be supported by Vint as the Anaesthetist and General Physician, and Di as the Ward Nurse and 'general dog's body.' Vint became an anaesthetist overnight after only three lessons from Penny, and I took over his position in the now well-established Pathology Laboratory.

In November the team left, heavily laden with operating tables, sterile packs and other equipment. Twenty-two porters were required to carry the necessities, in all about half a ton.

Yet even in that surprising country, nobody could have foreseen the dramatic circumstances of their arrival in Dankhutta: for on the trail they came across a woman of twenty-seven being carried on a litter, in the final stages of labour. She was in severe pain and the only chance she had to stay alive and to give birth was to reach a fully-equipped hospital. On John's advice the party turned round and within hours the Operating Theatre in Dankhutta was transformed and the patient brought to the table. A Caesarian Section was done and the mother was saved, as also was the baby, a son. This miraculous introduction opened the way for John and Vint as no calculated diplomacy could have done, and enabled them to establish themselves in a way from which future Trust Members were to benefit.

This first hill team had indeed a most difficult job to do. They had to gain the confidence of the local people whilst working under very primitive conditions. They also had to establish their own houses and adapt themselves to local customs and to the lack of amenities, not the least being the lack of running water and electricity. Water had to be collected from a pipe running down the village street and often the supply dwindled to a mere trickle. All cooking was done on a stove built from clay and the fumes from the wood-fire filtered through the house forcing one to open shutters to clear eyes of tears and rooms of swirling smoke. All four members of the team worked like beavers: FREQUENTLY Vint gave an anaesthetic and at the same time managed to do his daily quota of blood counts with his spare hand. Although this was only a preliminary advance into the unknown, the stage was set for a more permanent establishment in the future.

CHAPTER XII

Christmas in Nepal

When we left England, Penny had been three months pregnant — a fact which perhaps should have deterred us from attempting the journey at all; but we calculated that we had between us medical expertise and equipment enough to meet almost any emergency, and in the event she coped marvellously not only with the trip but with six months' work in the hospital afterwards.

So on November 18th 1968 our first son Andrew Sinclair was born in the British Military Hospital at Dharan at the ungodly hour of 5.30 a.m. From the beginning he was Andrew Sing to all our staff. We had always wanted a son and in Nepal a male first-born is counted a very good omen (a daughter is looked upon in a very different light).

Then our first Christmas was upon us. John and Sheena were to spend theirs in Calcutta, Vint and Di were off to the snow-covered hills of Darjeeling, and the rest of us had Christmas at home in Biratnagar.

Everyone pitched into preparations: we would make Christmas in Nepal as like as possible to Christmas at home. Barney somehow or other produced a Christmas tree; Penny had remembered to put our 'fairy lights' in our trunk; Peter's mother supplied a pudding and a cake; a turkey was suddenly promised from Dharan, and then there was Hank.

Hank, whom I have already mentioned, didn't take long becoming not only an ally of our team, but also a very popular friend. Within a few hours of the arrival of the first of our members in Biratnagar, he had been round at the house with offers of assistance. He also had the distinction of mixing the best Manhattans any of us had ever tasted and generally, after three, his stock was sky-high — as were the fortunate imbibers.

Hank invited us all to his house for Christmas Eve. His preparations were meticulous, and most of the day he stood in the kitchen with an apron round his middle, tending his Californian turkey. Rosemary went round to give him a hand, then we all gathered in his sitting room to listen to the Westminster Choir School singing carols, which he had taped on a visit to the U.K.

It was a real family dinner party, no refinement was forgotten, and it was well into Christmas morning before we went to bed.

Early on Christmas day Keith and Nigel, officers from Dharan, joined our party. Gill and Rosemary produced stockings packed with a wild assortment of oddities they had been able to scrounge from the bazaar during the previous week. Presents were distributed and Christmas post opened. We were delighted to find that many of our Nepalese friends had gone to the trouble to send us cards.

The day was not however to prove a holiday for Barney and me. There was an urgent call from the hospital, accompanied by profuse apologies for disturbing our holiday, to say that a seriously ill patient required a transfusion and, since no technicians were available, we were the only people who could make sure that the blood matched. Most of the day was spent in taking samples from volunteers until we found sufficient. When we got home we were tired and a little irritable. But the patient had survived.

The New Year saw the departure of Barney to the British Section of the East-West Highway, and by February Vint and John, Sheena and Di were on their way back to Dankhutta to work once again in the hospital.

CHAPTER XIII

Highway Interlude

During our seven weeks spent in Kathmandu with the British Ambassador we had met a great number of the people visiting or staying as guests in the Ambassador's Residence. Amongst these were two senior officials of the largest building organisation in the world, then known as the Ministry of Public Buildings and Works and now as the Department of the Environment. They were in Kathmandu to discuss the building of a section of highway in the Terai area of Western Nepal, as part of an Aid project which would eventually provide a highway from East to West across the country and form a section of the Trans-Asia Highway from Istanbul to the Malay Peninsula.

The British section was to be a seventy-five-mile stretch from Butwal in the West to the Narayani river in the East, and included a central hill section rising to two thousand five hundred feet. Other sections of the project were already under way, sponsored by India, the U.S.A. and the U.S.S.R., and when all is complete this complex will do a great deal to increase communication in Nepal and avoid long detours through India.

Quite naturally the question of medical facilities cropped up and after considerable discussion it was agreed that we should put forward plans for medical coverage on the Highway, and that we should second a member of our team to work there on a six-month rotating basis. The Department would gain from the fact that they would have a resident doctor with a knowledge of the country and its people, and we would be providing a much-needed service for three thousand workers and their families.

Out came the paper and pencils to estimate the requirements of a General Practice which would eventually stretch for nearly eighty miles and include not only fifty expatriate staff and some wives, but also three thousand locally employed workers and their families.

The Base Camp was to be established near Butwal and was to be of a semi-permanent nature, and further camps would be built as the road progressed. At Base we certainly required a well-equipped Hospital and for this hospital we would need auxiliary staff. Forward medical posts would be required with which contact would be maintained by radio, and an ambulance.

The first small party of British staff arrived from the United Kingdom in October 1968 and Barney left to join them on January 1st 1969. Once again he was landed with a most difficult job, which he tackled with his usual energy. The Base Camp at this time consisted of a small clearing hacked out of dense jungle. His accommodation was half a tent and his surgery the other half, so that to get into bed he had to leap over the packing cases which served him as a desk. Then the usual difficulties arose from a hold-up of equipment in Bombay Docks. Food was difficult to obtain; and the water supply was inadequate and contaminated, producing the inevitable cases of dysentery.

Plans were made for the building of the hospital, and indeed this was the first building to be finished. Ex-Gurkha medical orderlies were recruited through the army base at Paklihawa, and a training programme started to prepare them for the time when they would be working by themselves at advance camps. Living quarters were being built meanwhile, as the first section of road was being carved out of the jungle.

Barney even found time to start a snake collection, by the simple expedient of offering one rupee (five new pence) for each foot of snake delivered to the surgery. Now most snakes in Nepal are small and only three are deadly poisonous: the cobra, the krait and the Himalayan pit viper. But one day appeared a gang of workers towing through the camp the largest of the Nepali snakes, a fourteen-foot python. This offering presented Barney with a problem, for apart from the fact that it would cost him no less than fourteen rupees, he worked out that he would need forty gallons of spirit in which to keep it. So, regretfully, he had to refuse it. It was towed on its way, no doubt to be eaten, for python is treated as a delicacy in Nepal.

Obtaining fresh water was a pressing problem, not only for the expatriate staff, but particularly for the workers whose only supply was from the polluted stream close to the camp. Drill holes were started but no water could be found in the immediate area, until by chance a soil-drilling rig just over a mile away encountered water at only fifty feet. Samples sent for culture proved it to be drinkable and pipes were laid to carry it to the camp area.

Butwal was at least ten degrees hotter than Biratnagar and as it was surrounded by jungle, little air filtered into the camp. The extreme heat of May and early June produced inevitable cases of heatstroke, and by the time I took over from Barney in June 1969 we were longing for the monsoon to break. When the first major storm did come, however, it nearly resulted in catastrophe. The howling wind tore down a number of giant trees which crashed upon several buildings in the immediate area. Shaken but fortunately unhurt, British engineers crawled from their rooms to survey the damage. The following morning several more trees toppled, this time felled by nimble Nepalis who are expert in judging the direction of fall to avoid damage.

The monsoon brought with it further difficulties. The access track soon became a morass, and work at the advance camps had to be suspended almost completely. Many of the locally employed staff were hillmen, Gurungs and Magars from the Western Hills, Limbus and Rais from the East, and with the arrival of the monsoon and the drop in demand for their labour, many workers returned to their homes.

Across the road from the base camp a new village had sprung up and soon a school was opened for the children, a venture that was actively supported by the U.K. staff. When the road is completed there will be several similar villages along its routes, and already enterprising Nepalis were looking for land on which to open small hotels and garages.

The medical orderlies led by Bhoj Bahadur Gurung all turned out to be very willing to learn. It soon became apparent that they would be quite capable of taking care of most, if not all, immediate first aid problems, from the treatment of minor injuries to the care of more serious cases until they could be transferred by ambulance to hospital. Surprisingly we had few accidents during the first year although minor injuries were common. And I could not have asked for a better ambulance driver. Safe at all times, he certainly holds the record from the base camp to the foot of the Hill Section. Admiring engineers remarked that he was airborne when he passed them with an urgent case. The one-way journey normally took two hours — he did the return journey in less than three in an emergency.

To build seventy-five miles of road sounds a fairly simple problem. But to build a road over Nepali Terai terrain is an unpredictable business at the best of times. Dense jungle and water-logged rice fields are pierced by dozens of streams which within half-an-hour can become raging torrents. Rivers flowing placidly in the dry season will flood to ten times their normal width when the rains come. The Hill Section had to be hacked out of mud and rock and protected from damage by landslides. Thousands of trees had to be hewn down and their roots torn out, and culverts built at intervals of two hundred yards to cope with drainage. Out ahead of the main gangs went the surveyors, protected by armed policemen from the occasional tiger whose jungle liberty might be threatened. Behind came the bulldozers and the earthmovers, the dumpers and the stone crushers, the men and the women who fashion the road.

Back at base the Quantity Surveyors juggled with figures and the Catering Officer received his daily quota of grouses and grumbles. Lee Campbell had been in charge of catering almost since the road started and he provided excellent food under extraordinary conditions: it is very difficult to please fifty people who come from very different areas of the country and whose ideas of what is suitable to eat can be extremely various. 'Salmon again?' one could hear muttered from a corner. 'No chips with the curry?' from another. At least at Christmas no complaint was heard when the spread rivalled the Savoy in substance as well as in quantity.

A Pub, inevitably called 'The Highwayman', was the central meeting point for nearly all, and Friday night was the time to let one's hair down before the weekly day-off on Saturday. The way back to the living quarters was often indistinct but most people made it, notably Reg, the surveyor, who was celebrated for pursuing a dead-straight line across flower beds and through monsoon drains without more than half-a-degree departure from his course.

CHAPTER XIV

Patients

The immense physical courage of the Nepalese people has for long been something of a legend; and their uncomplaining ability to withstand terrible injuries, their patient endurance of disease is a subject of which I have now some personal knowledge.

Only a few weeks after our arrival in Nepal a young hill man was admitted to the British Military Hospital in Dharan with half his face torn away in a fight with a wild bear. In this condition he had walked for six days to the hospital. where he remained for many months undergoing plastic surgery. He never complained — he accepted his condition as the 'luck of the draw'. Another had been tending his goats when a leopard had attacked the flock. Armed with a *kukri,* he took on the leopard and succeeded in killing it, nearly losing an arm in the process.

Many people will walk for days with an acute abdominal emergency which would have been treated by immediate operation in Europe. Their life is always hard and in illness they display the same fortitude as they do in health.

Yet while on the one hand the Nepalese can show this incredible will to live, on the other, a patient may simply resolve to die. If this happens, there is very little the doctor can do about it, except wait for the inevitable conclusion. This seemingly inexplicable power of the will has been witnessed by several Europeans.

To lose a leg, or even worse the right hand, is often such a catastrophe that the patient will ask to die. A healthy young man was admitted to hospital after he had been hunting in the jungle. He had picked up a small ball-like object, illegally used for killing wild boar, and, like a grenade, it exploded in his hands, tearing them to shreds. The look of horror on his face when he fully realised the extent of his injuries, arose not from the thought of the injuries themselves, but from the fear that he had lost all means of supporting his family. Fortunately skilful surgery saved more than we had first imagined possible, and his relief knew no bounds.

Quack doctors still flourish in many areas of the country, though fortunately belief in them is dying out as the interest in Western medicine spreads. Cataracts in the eye are still treated by the barbaric means of displacing the lens by the use of a thorn — resulting in immediate temporary improvement and then often in glaucoma and complete painful blindness. Cow-dung is applied to wounds, to disinfect them — and produces tetanus (lock-jaw). Garlic is tied to limbs to reduce swelling — and often burns through to the bone. The illegal midwives who assist with labours often cause death to a mother by mismanagement, or produce tetanus in a baby by using a dirty knife to cut the cord.

Foul-selling concoctions are sold in the streets as cures for all ills. For stomache-ache you drink them, for rheumatism you rub them on, and I doubt if there is a use to which you cannot put them. I am also quite certain that they do not one atom of good.

On the other hand every tribal group has its own tested traditional remedies, carried down from generation to generation. A large Limbu porter showed me with great glee how to cure my amoebic dysentery by drinking the juice from a small red fruit. I regret to say that the taste was so terrible that I couldn't keep it down. And most efficient splints are made from the sap of a creeper, which sets hard in the sun. We saw more and more examples of simple but effective treatments for common disorders the longer we stayed in the country. Perhaps Nepal will yet supply a medical product as valuable as *curare,* the South American arrow poison now widely used in anaesthetics.

Death in childbirth is very common, even in hospital, for Nepalese mothers seem subject to every form of complication of pregnancy known to medicine, most of them rarely seen in the U.K. Some mothers are so anaemic that they cannot sit unaided. Small mothers, whose bone structure will not allow them to give birth to their child, arrive exhausted after many days in labour. But gradually, with increased ante-natal care, mortality will fall.

The lot of the newly born infant is probably even worse. Only six or seven out of every ten will be alive at the end of the first year. The rest are carried off by dysentery, tetanus, chest infections, tuberculosis and malnutrition, to mention but a few of nature's ravages.

Our first problem, then, was often one of communication — we had to gain the co-operation of our patients, somehow to get them to understand what we were doing, and why. From the beginning there was a clear distinction between the attitudes of Out-Patients and In-Patients, for the Out-Patients department was always thronged with people eager for treatment, whereas once in the wards, their demeanour seemed to change. They were frequently bewildered, scared, unable to understand what was happening to them, and feeling cut off from homes and relatives — who in turn would add to the confusion by hanging round the beds, pestering doctors and nurses in their efforts to comprehend prognosis and treatment, or simply languishing, mystified but too frightened to ask.

Yet we had so little time to stop, and make the effort necessary even to begin to bridge the immense gap between their experience and ours. On the whole, we had to rely on our practical successes to gain the trust we required. For the hospital was always full to overflowing, we often had beds set up in the corridors, and accident cases and burns frequently blocked the beds so that urgent surgical cases or serious medical cases were barred from the wards simply for lack of beds. Accidents abounded, especially in the mango season when numerous small boys would break their legs falling out of fruit trees; and road accidents were always plentiful.

I remember an Indian who had been in a lorry accident, presumably delivering goods from India, who had fractured the upper leg, so that the femur had broken through the skin. The wound was sutured and the bone set in a hurry, partly because there were so many other injured to deal with that day, partly because he was bleeding copiously. Then, a couple of days later he began to show symptoms of gas gangrene, a highly infectious condition which spreads very quickly. His leg would have to be amputated. This necessitated a tremendous upheaval because it could not be done in the theatre, for risk of the germs remaining behind and infecting following cases, so we had to use a little side room, and all the equipment had to be wheeled through. The poor man's spirit was virtually shattered by the loss of his leg and he didn't do at all well, until one day, when it had been healing satisfactorily, we decided to try and boost his morale by bringing in our driver to make him a crutch. This he did with great success, and the change in the man's attitude was marvellous. He started to get up and about, and later on we were able to send him to Dharan to the military hospital where an artificial limb was made for him, a crude object very much like the peg-leg of Long John Silver, nothing like modern artificial limbs, but nevertheless enough to restore him to the sense of being a man able to work and earn his own living.

Burns were another big problem and some of the burns sustained by women especially were horrifying, since once a sari catches fire it flares up like a roman candle. And it is the women of course who bend over open fires and kerosene stoves. We had one very brave little girl (little, though she must have been about twenty-three years of age) who had extensive burns on her body, and on occasions her shouts and screams when they were being dressed were heart-rending. Yet she soldiered on, when I think most

English-women in the same condition would have died, with her father to support her, for he hardly left her side. She survived until one day he had to bring her the news that her husband had taken a new wife. This was the end. She just gave up, eventually discharged herself, and we must presume that she died.

Maternity cases were varied and frequently very dramatic. And even when no medical complications arose, there were sometimes social ones. One Muslim lady, for instance, had to have a womb 'scrape' postponed for days, while she bled quite dangerously, because her husband and her father were adamant that no man should be in theatre for such an intimate operation. They prowled around the hospital until we could give them an absolute guarantee that no man would be in there. She could in the long run possibly have bled to death; but luckily we had a woman surgeon and with Penny as anaesthetist the operation was done.

On another occasion, over a Nepali religious festival, we were on duty without the Nepalese staff, so I had to stitch up a girl after she had been cut for delivery. She was a well-educated girl and spoke very good English, but she persisted in practising her English on me throughout the operation, although she was clearly deeply embarrassed by having the British Sahib stitch her up, and came back regularly to the Children's Clinic and told all the other mothers about it. She was one of those who thought it clever to overfeed her baby and the poor little chap became a real Michelin man. But he was always clean and never suffered from the tummy bugs that so many of the children used to get.

The Clinics were for mothers and babies, well ones as well as ill ones, such as had already been established in many areas of the country. When we first arrived the place was a miracle of clamour and disorder, but gradually we managed to get the Nepali nurses to organise themselves. We had one and sometimes two doctors examining the children, and it was very gratifying to see the improvement

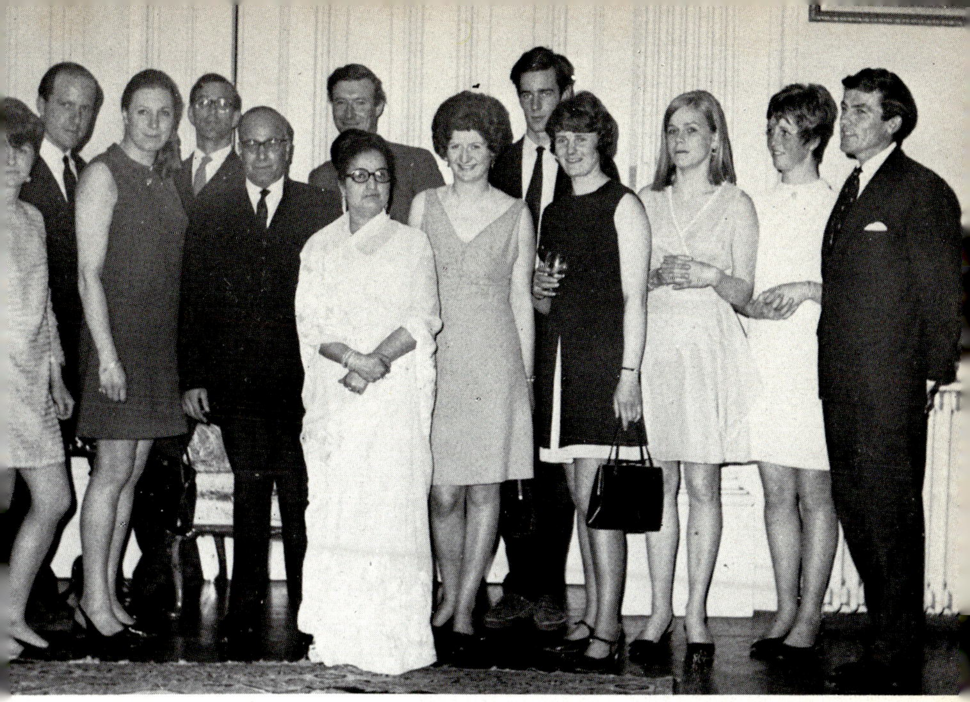

1. The Team before setting off for Nepal, at a reception given by the Royal Nepalese Embassy, London. l to r Di, Vint, Penny, Barney, His Excellency the Ambassador, his wife, John Cunningham, Rosemary, Peter, Gill, Sheena, Prue, John Ward

2. The signing of the contract at Sinha Durba, Kathmandu. Centre are John Ward, John Cunningham, and Dr. Das, Director of Health Services. Photo: *Information Service, H M Government, Nepal*

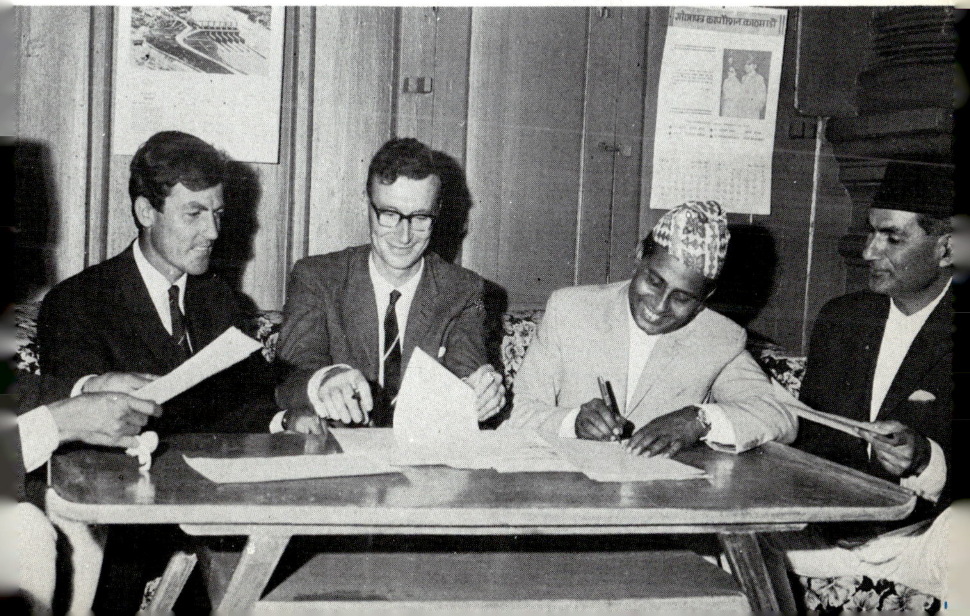

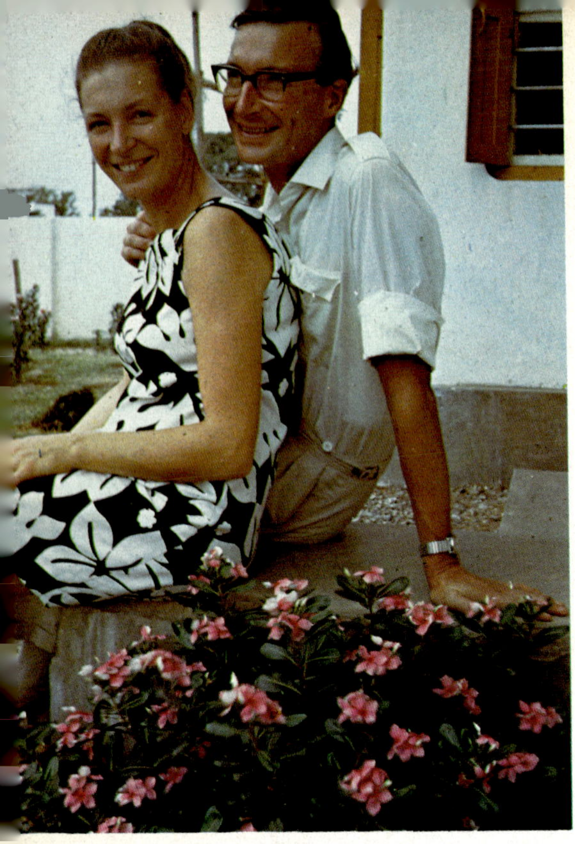

3. The author and his wife, Penny, at their home in Nepal

4. The Raj Path — the road to Kathmandu

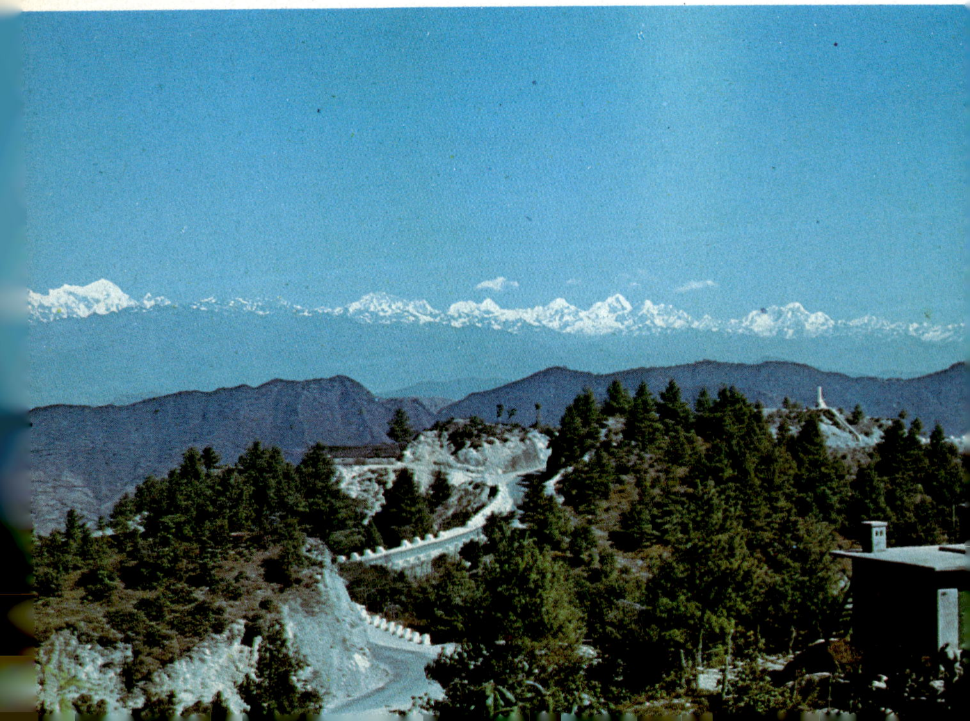

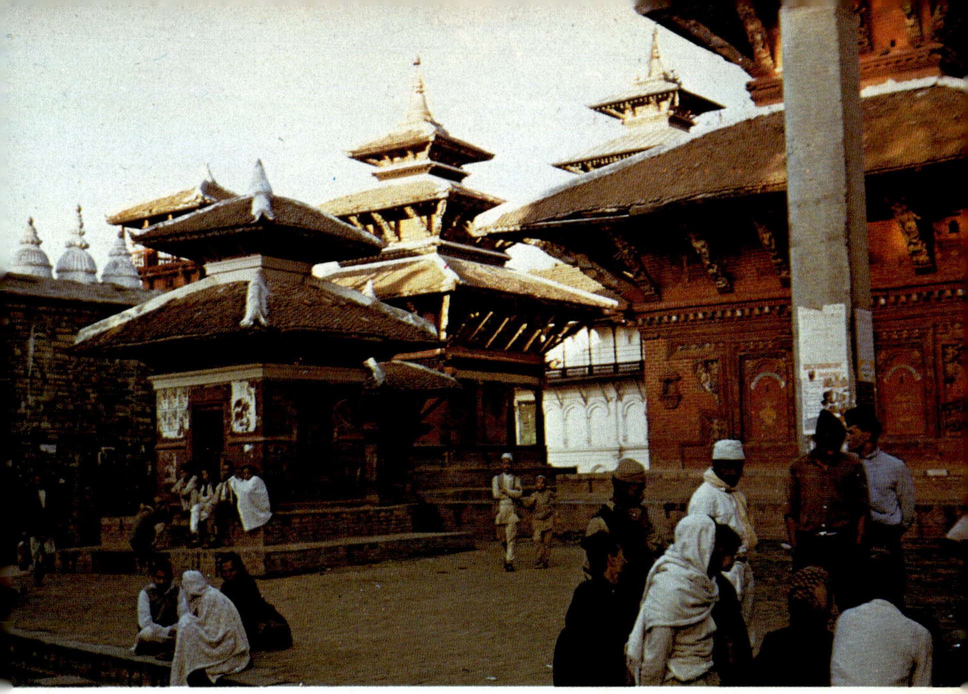

5. Durbar Square, Kathmandu

6. Kathmandu

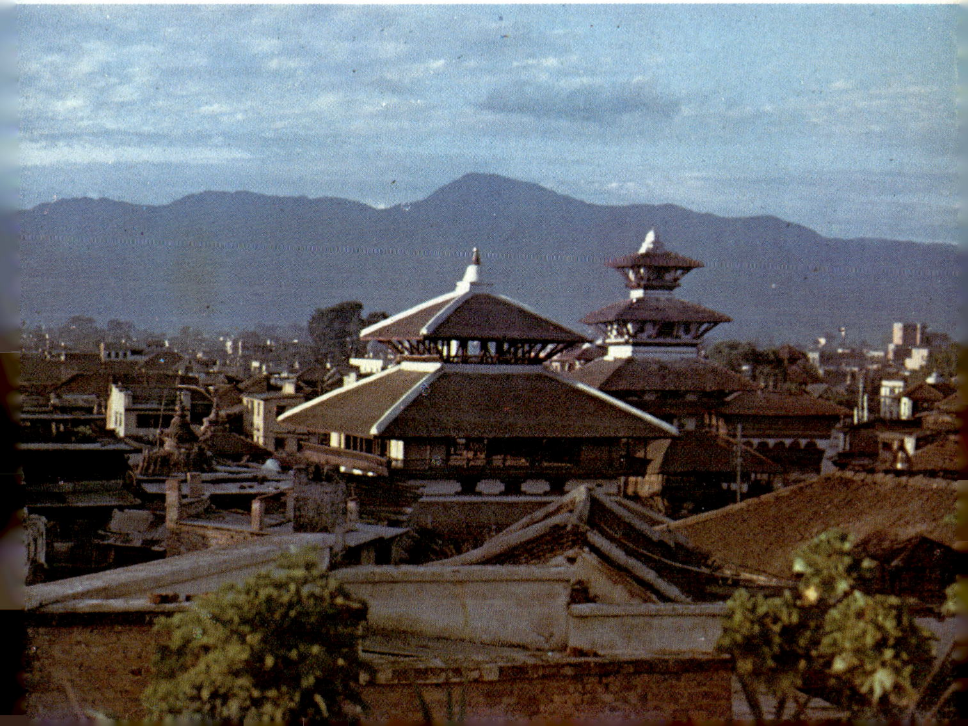

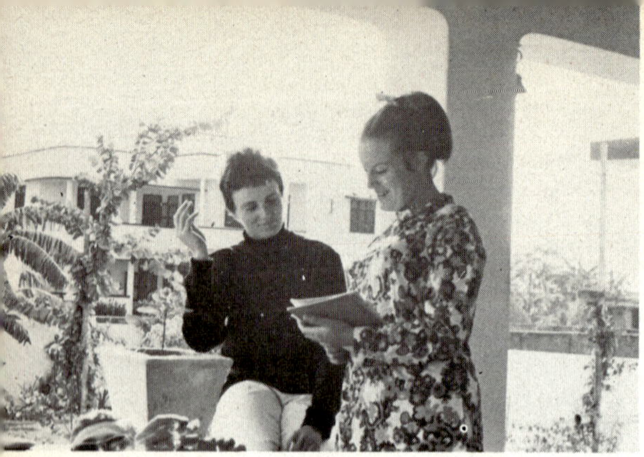

7. Gill and Hilary — Kafle Nivas in the background

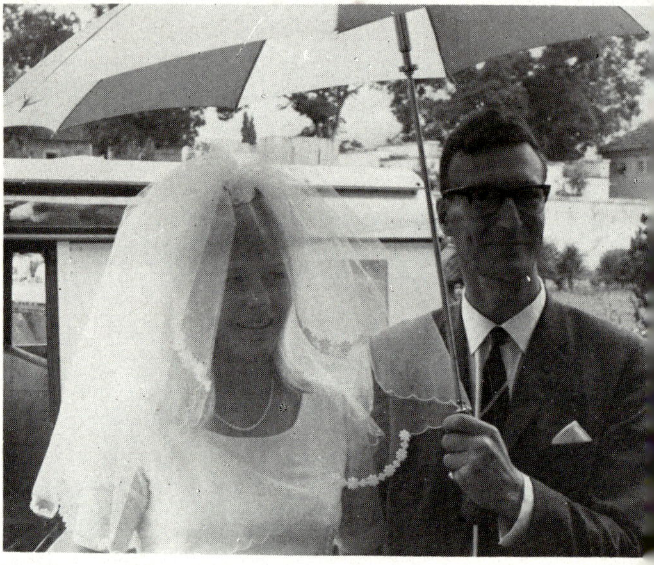

8. Giving the bride away — Sheena and the author

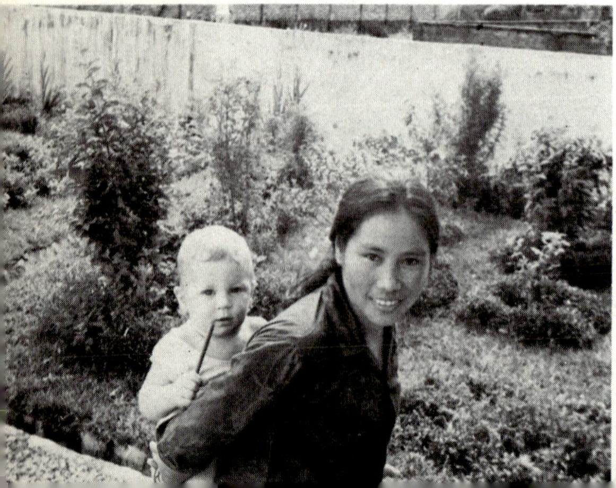

9. Andrew with his *ayah*, Bishnu

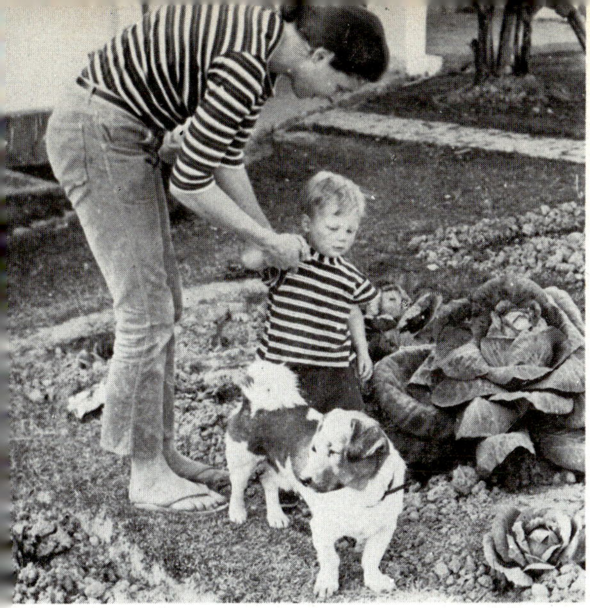

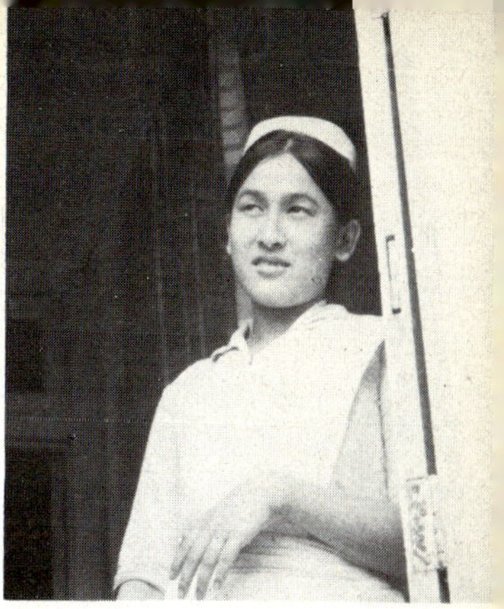

11. Nepali nurse

10. Penny, Andrew and Makalu

12. Outside Kafle Nivas

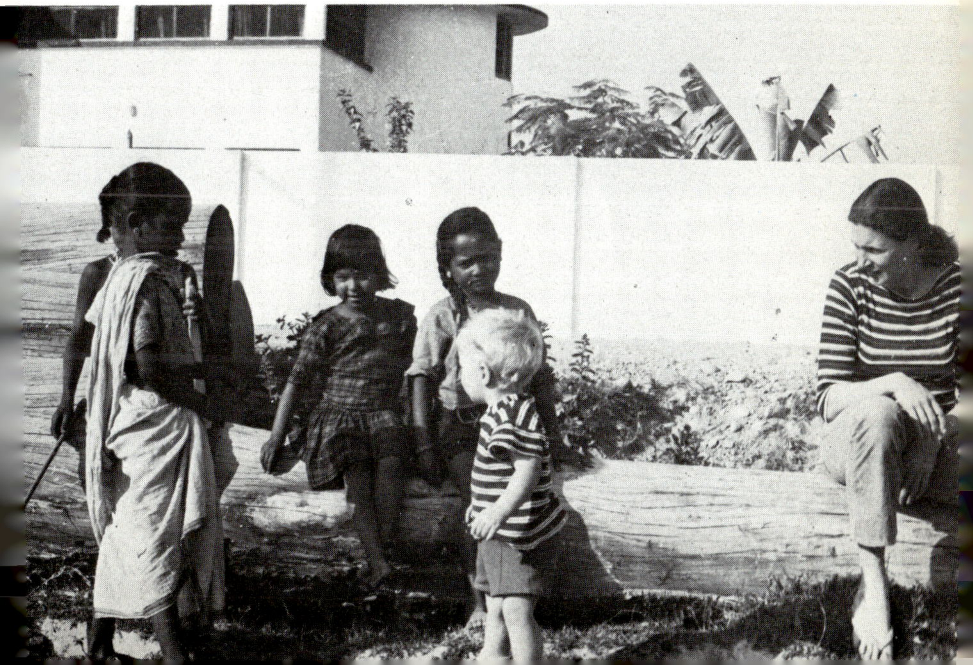

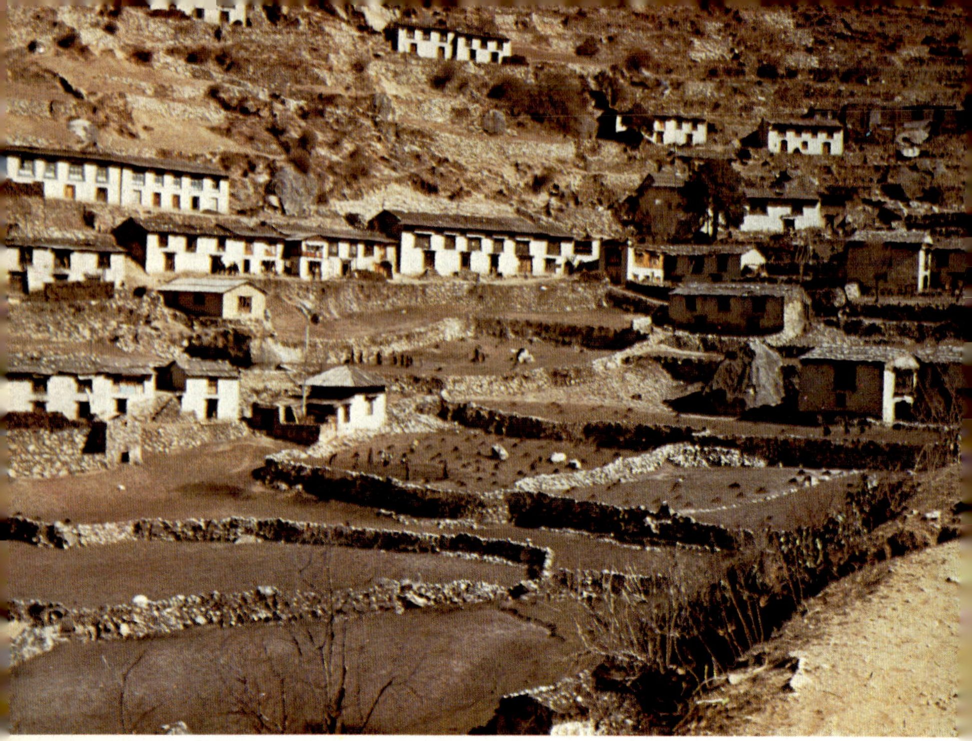

13. The village of Namche Bazaar

14. Dankhutta Hospital

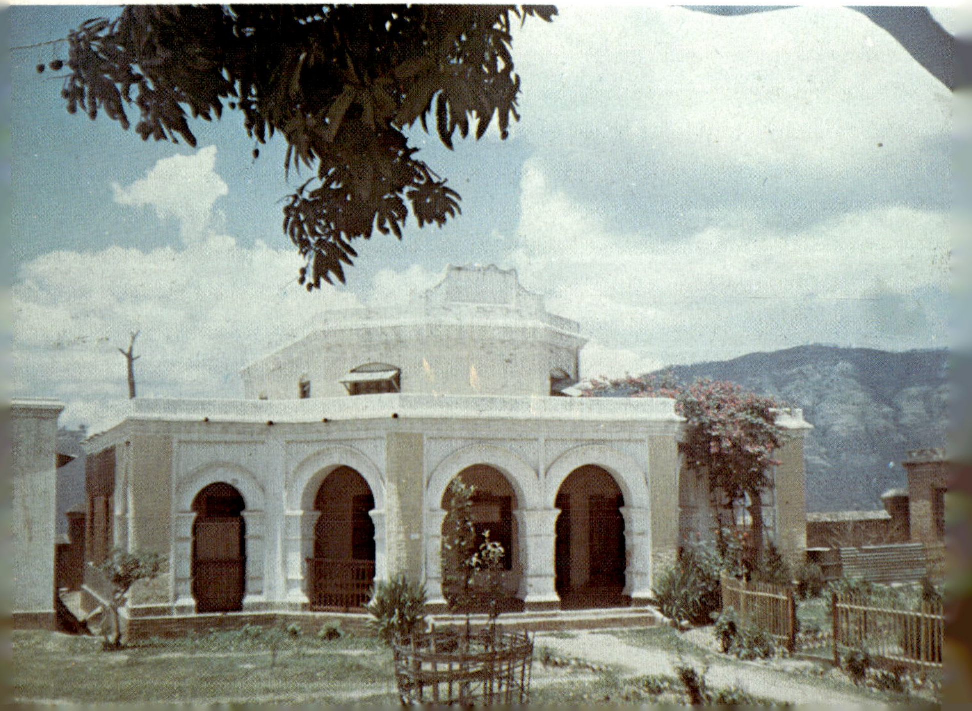

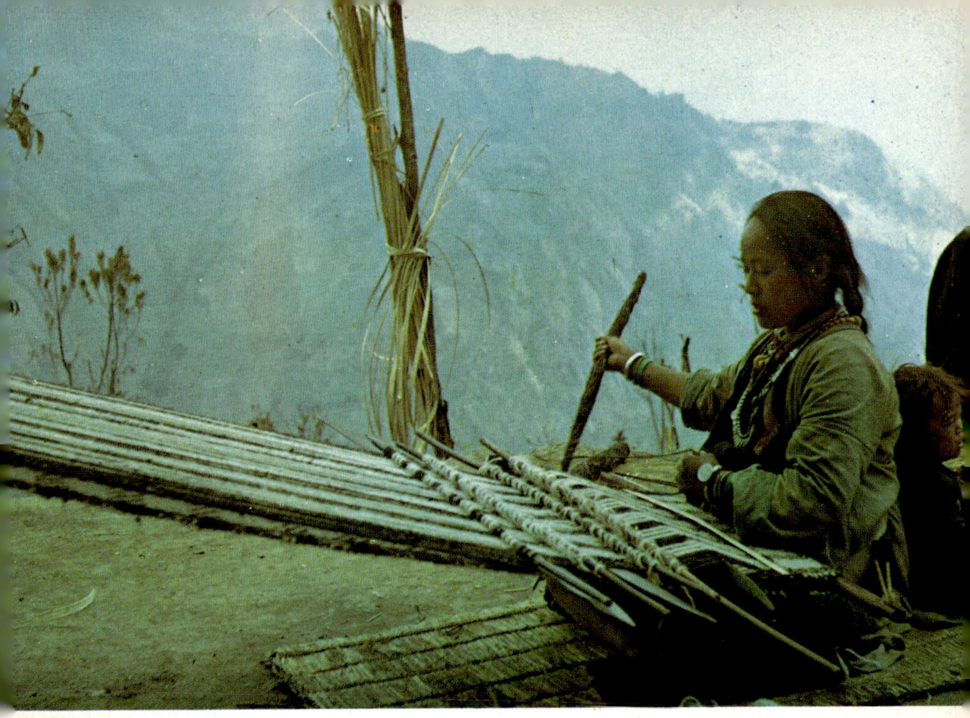

15. A Sherpa girl weaving

16. Hill people

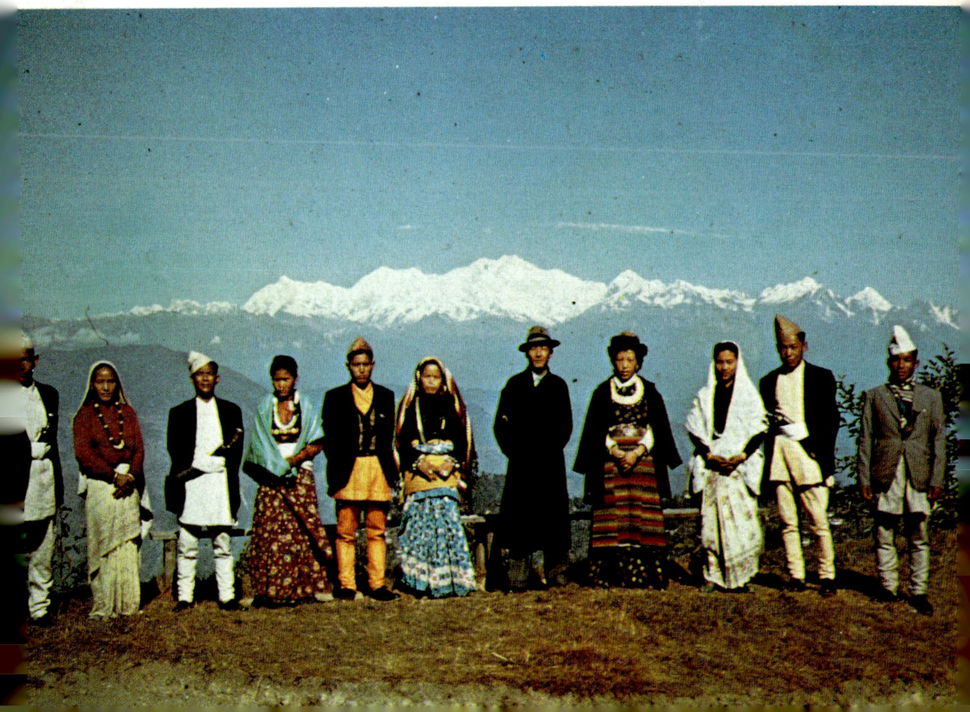

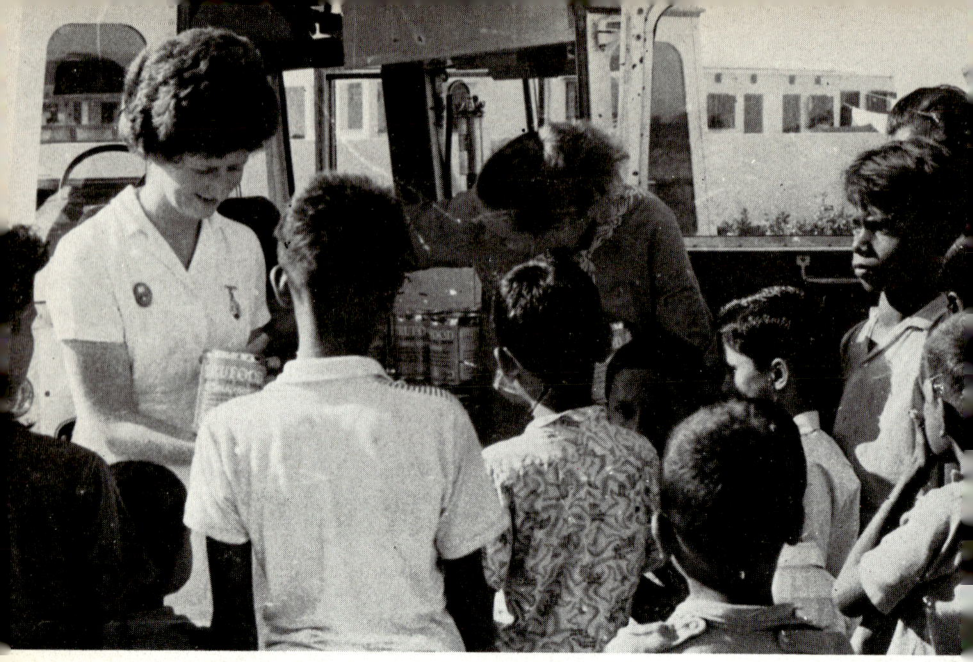

17. The BCG team at work

18. Old woman at Sun Baluwa

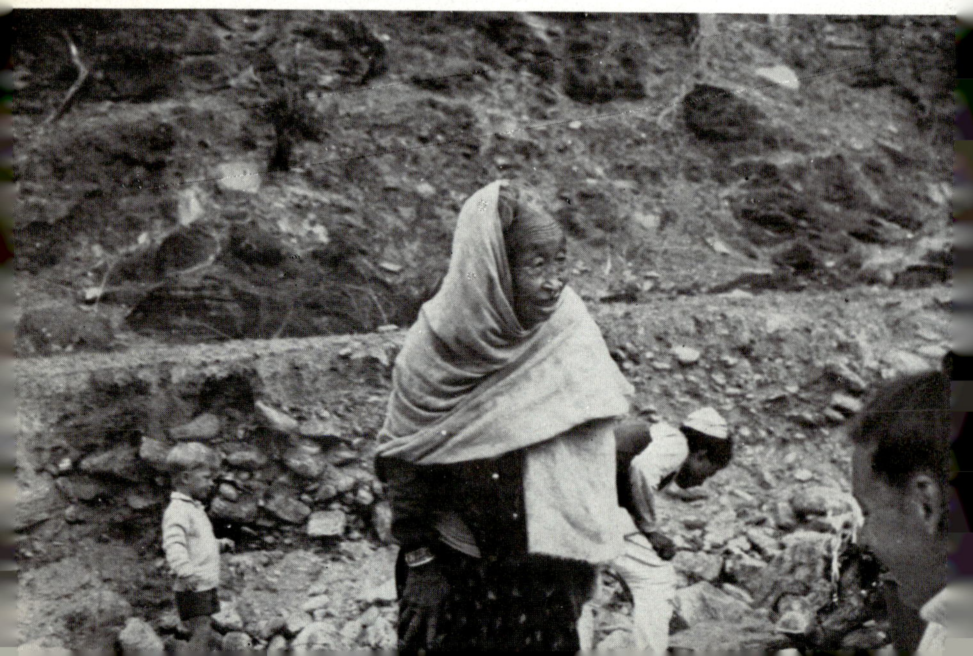

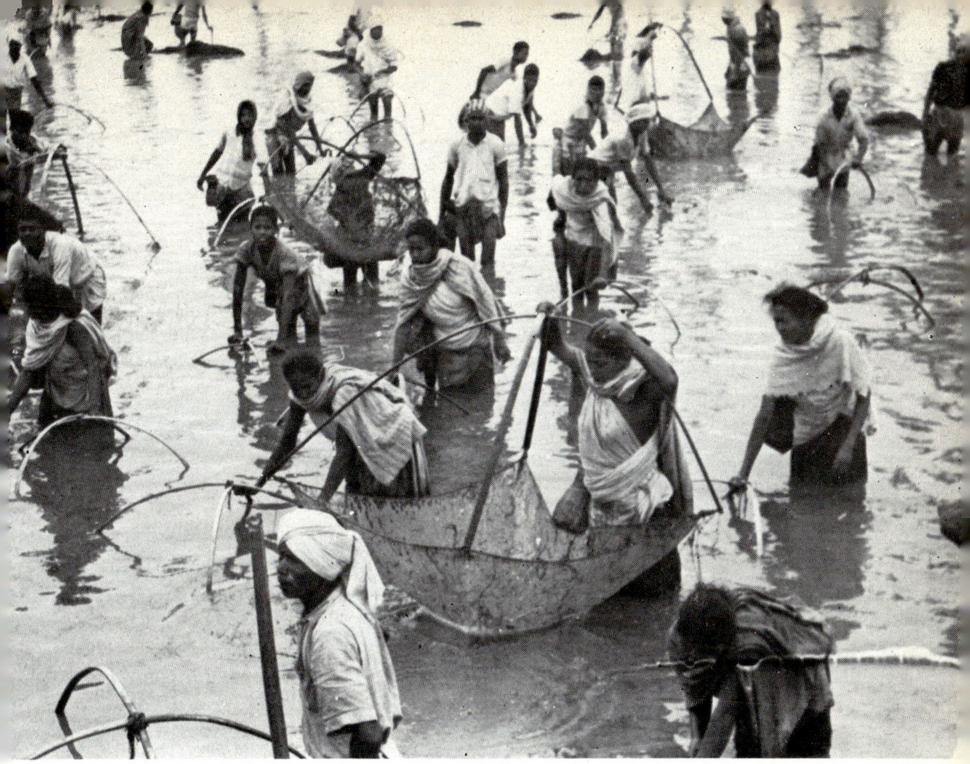

19. Fishermen in the Terai

20. The Fish-Tail Lodge, Pokhara

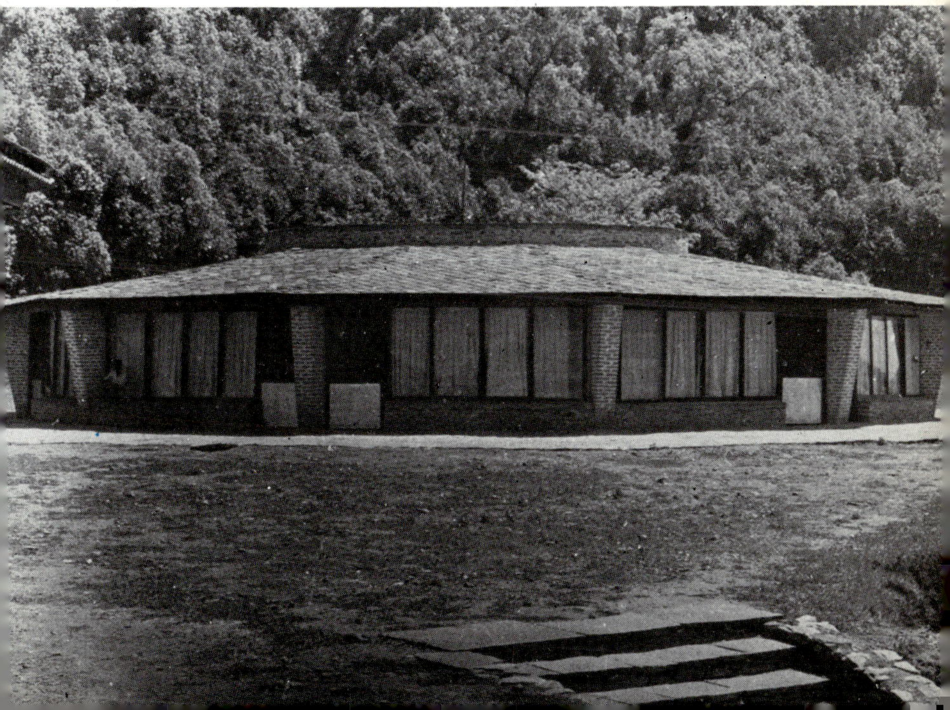

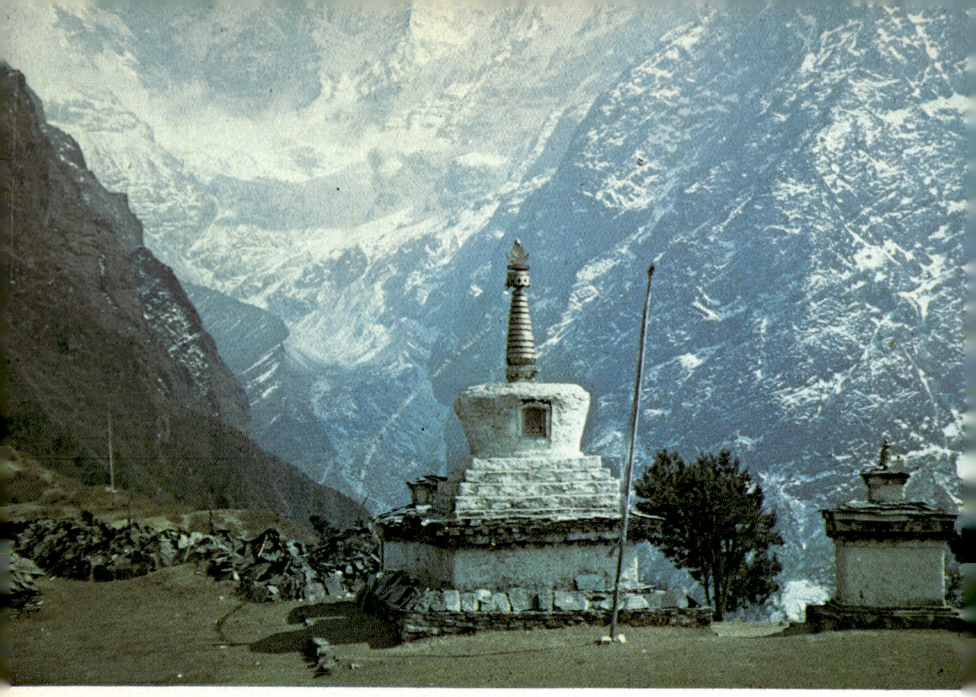

21. A Stupa, or Bhuddist shrine, at Namche

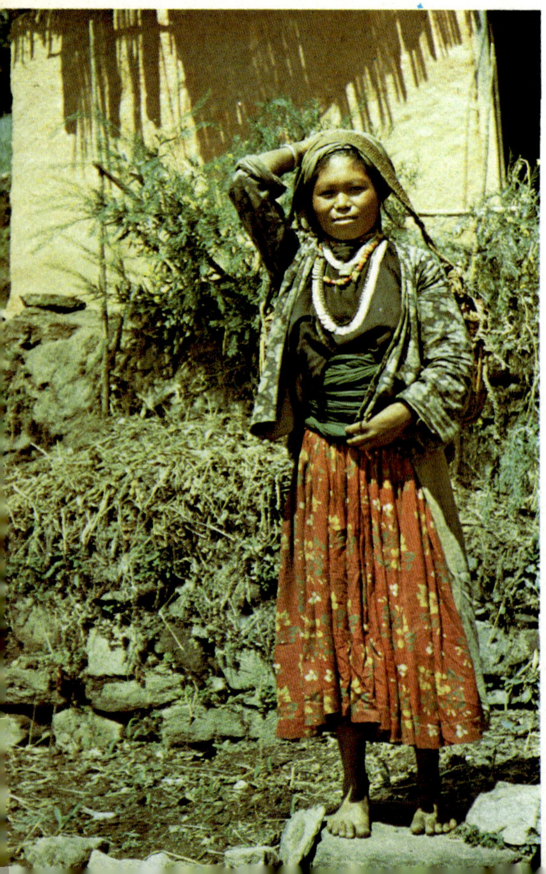

22. Sherpa girl

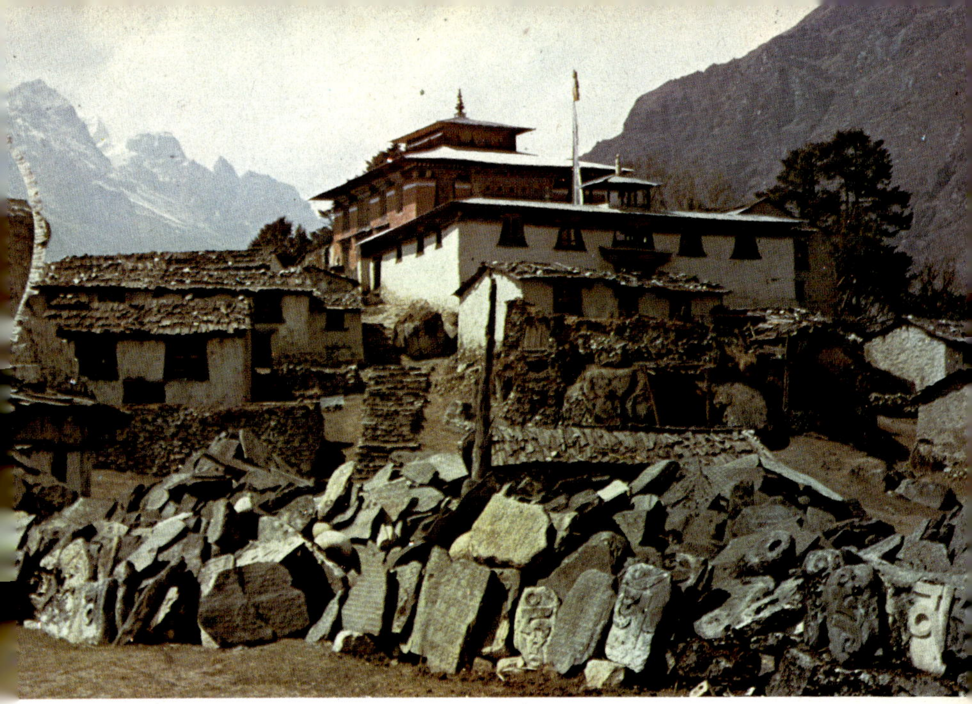

23. Tang Boche Monastery, high on the way to Everest

24. Chainpur

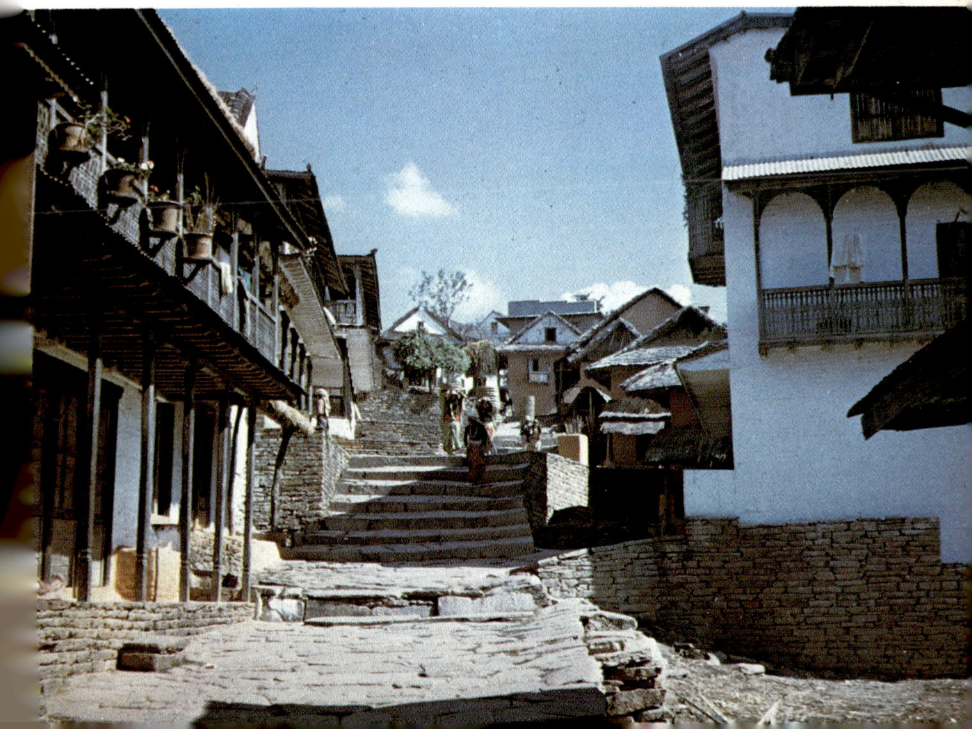

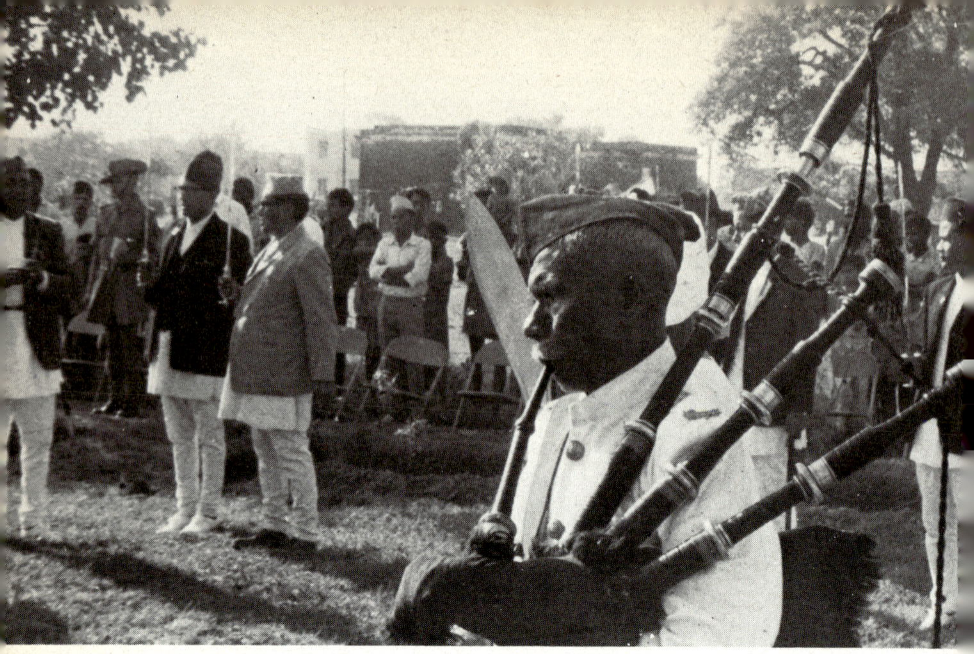

25. Royal Nepalese Army piper at Hindu festival in Butwal

26. Prem Bahadur, our original bearer, on trek

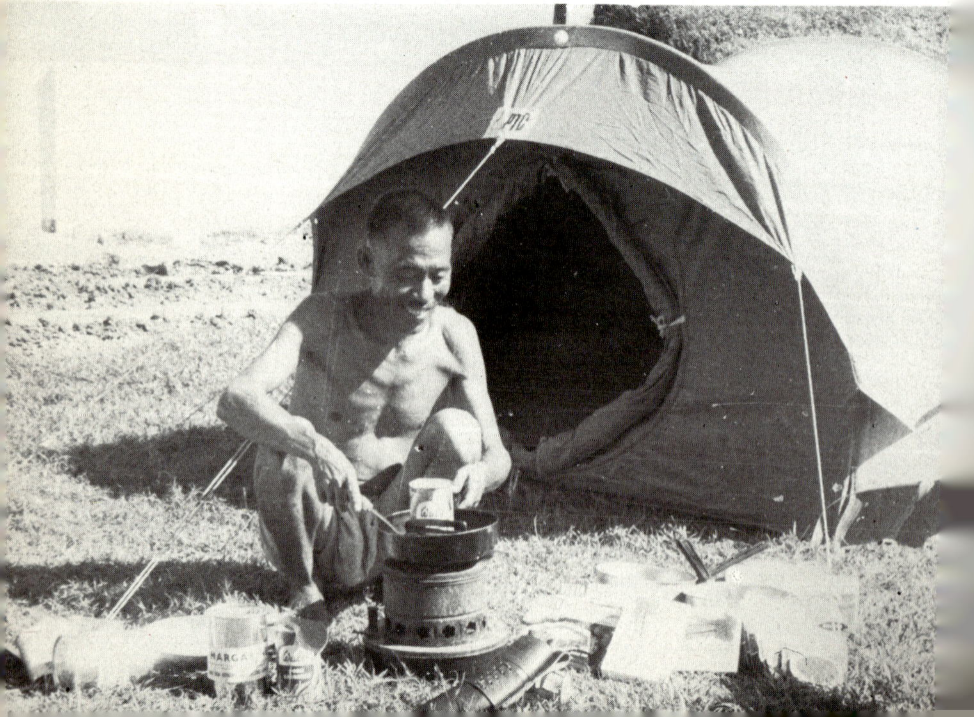

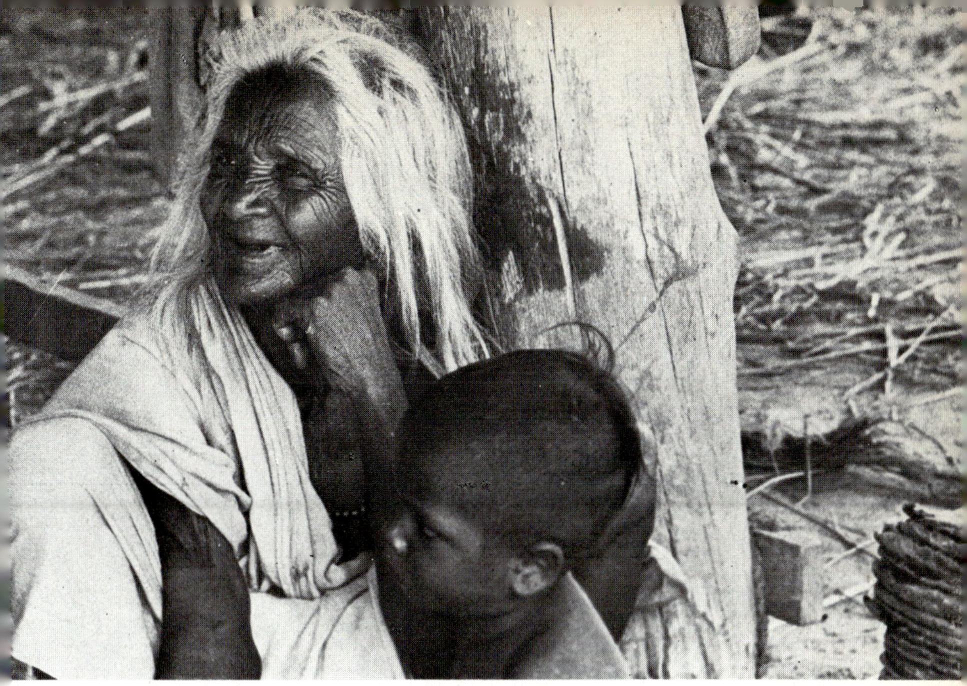

27, 28. Nepalese faces

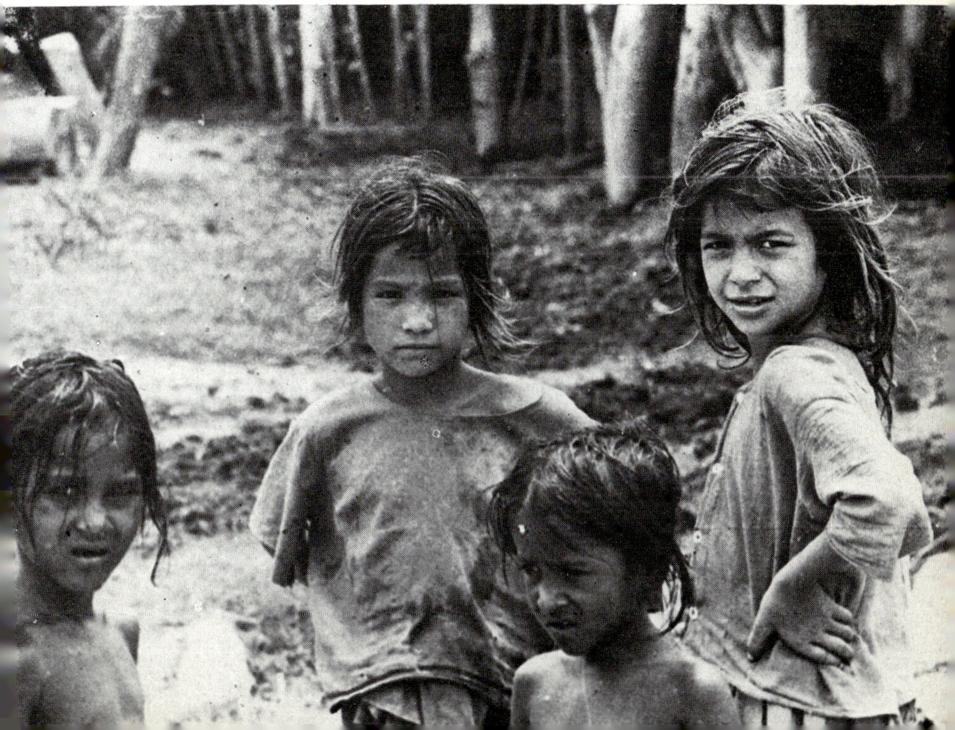

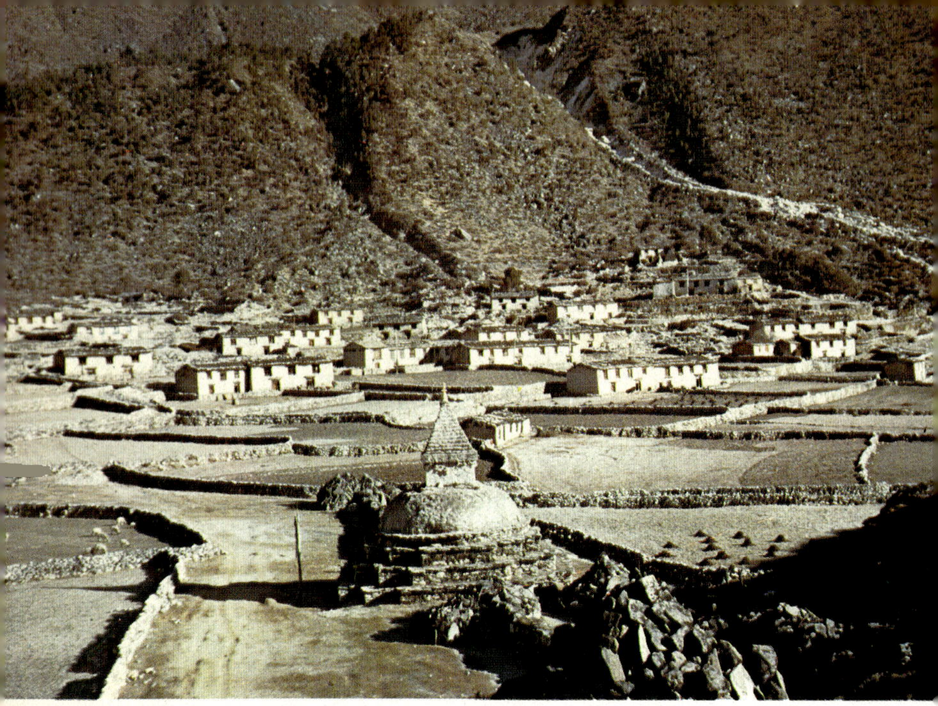

29. The village of Kunde

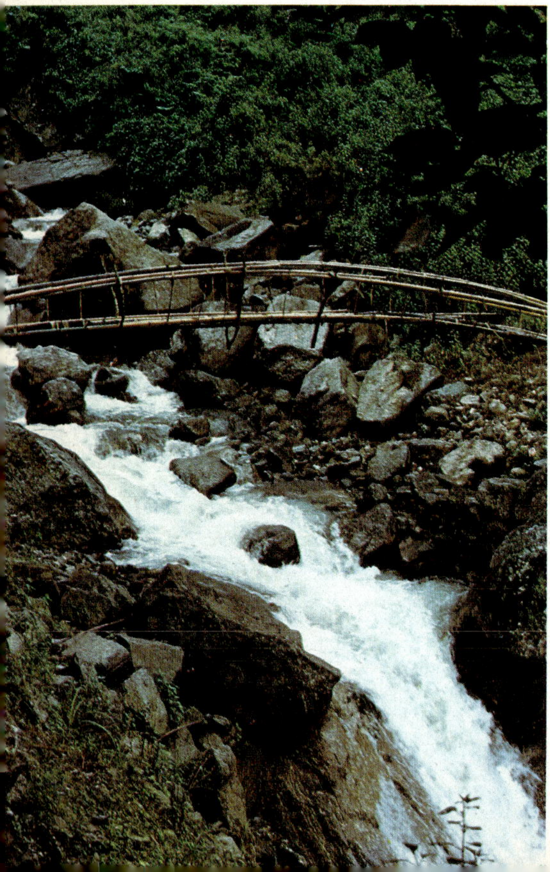

30. Footbridge — the river below is sometimes a torren

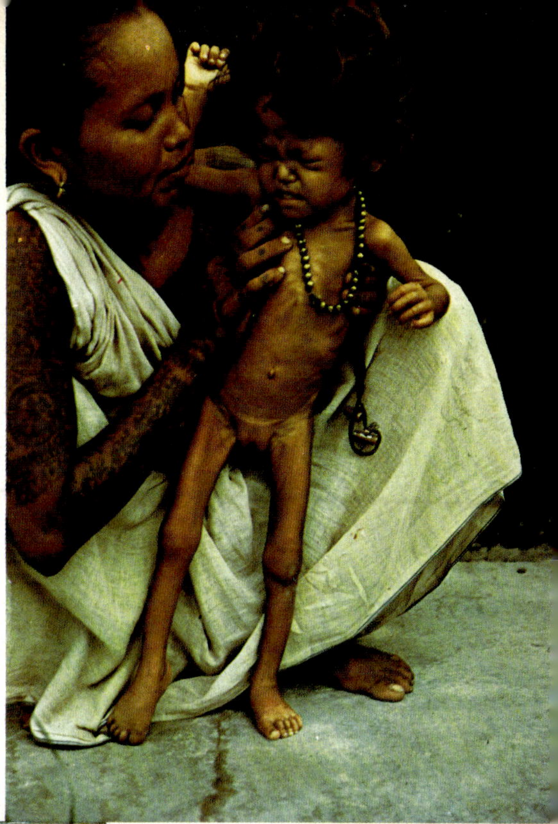

31. Extreme malnutrition

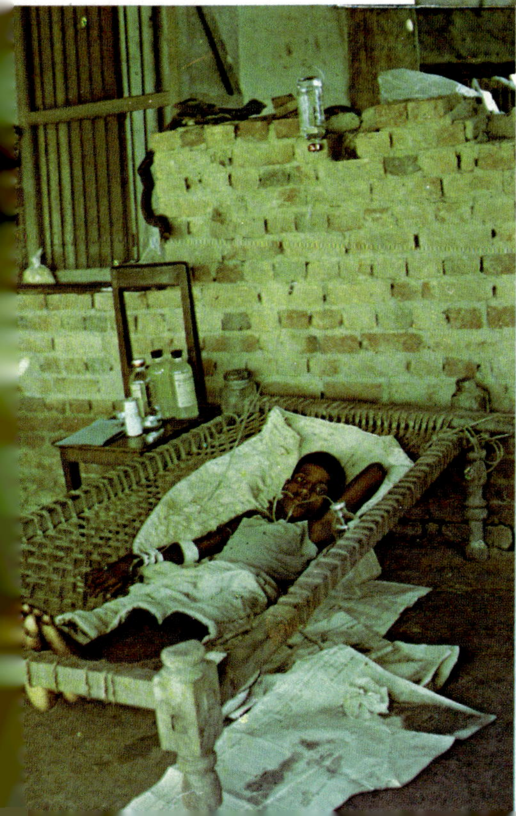

32. A cholera patient

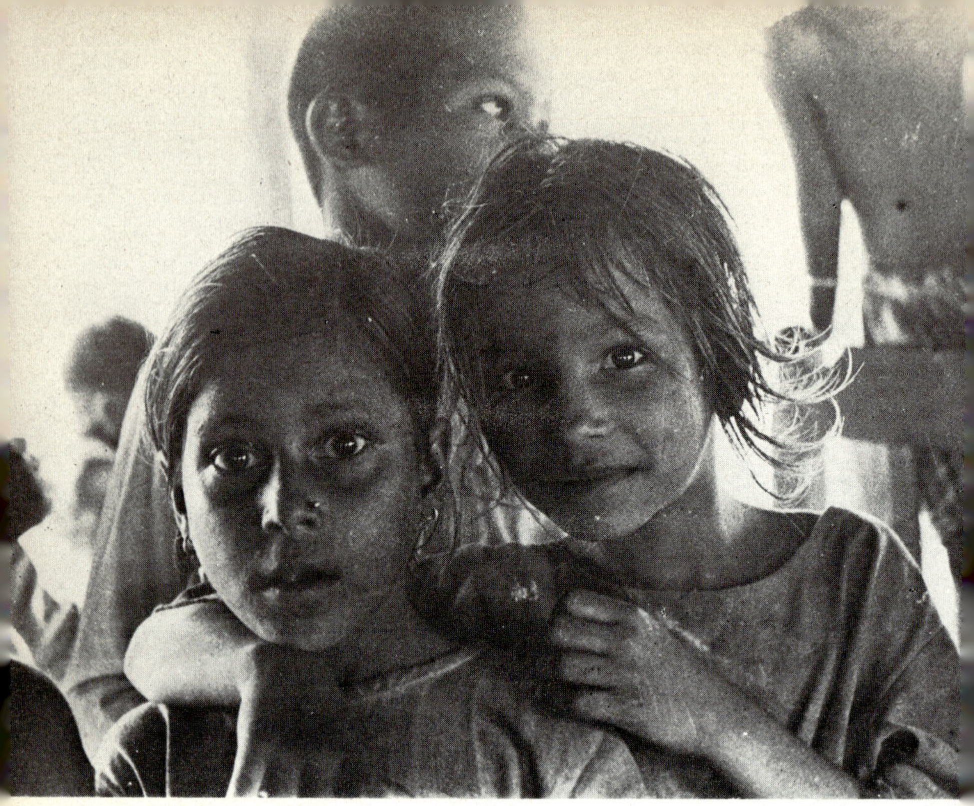

33. Nepalese faces

34 At the foot of the Ice Giant

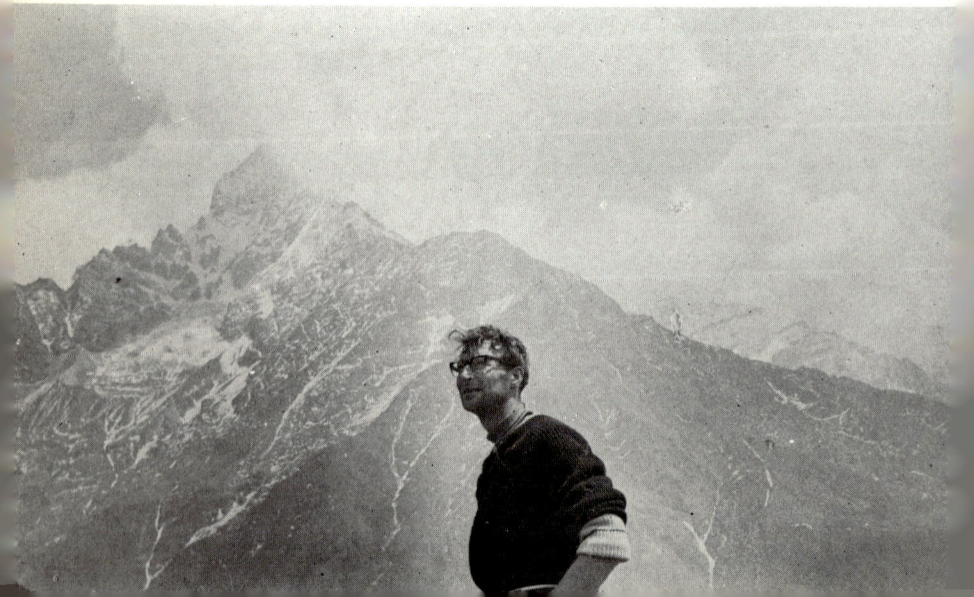

in many of the children over the first year or so. Our aim was to make sure that they were adequately nourished, that they were as free from disease as possible and that those in real need received extra milk and extra vitamins. We were not always able to supply these — sometimes we were short of drugs, sometimes we were short of milk — but somehow or other we always managed to give something. We were able to note progress even after the first year, for many people who had come first in a sceptical frame of mind, were still coming, pleased and happy to show off their children, dressing them up for the occasion, and dressing themselves in their best saris. Nepali nurses knelt on the floor showing mothers how to cook rice, or dahl (lentils), and preserve the nutrients, and after the cooking, of course, all the children gathered around in great glee to eat it all up. Milk they gulped down as if it was the best thing they had tasted in their lives — it was quite a sight.

Since Penny had made her first appearance in Nepal five months pregnant, and the whole town knew when Andrew was born, she had a special status in the children's clinic. The mothers, knowing that she was a mother herself, were willing to listen to her. One small girl of two-and-a-half or three had reason to be grateful for this: she was the victim of second-baby disease, that is, she had been literally pushed off the breast when another baby came along, forced to eat normal food with no preparation in a normal weaning process, and she just didn't like it. Since the parents were very poor and uneducated, they were unable to afford special and tempting foods for her, so when she was presented in the clinic she was in a shocking state, with skinny arms and legs and a very swollen abdomen, like one of the Oxfam babies. She was admitted, and proceeded to scream from morning to night. Most of the Nepali girls love children and are very good with them, but even their patience was tried with this little one. Luckily, we had with us at the time an American nurse sent by the World Health Organisation on a tour of three months at each of the major hospitals round the country. Her task was to advise on a scheme for training student nurses on the wards rather than in the classroom. She was a delightful, very extroverted girl and all the Nepali nurses liked her, so she took it upon herself to help them help this baby. After a very short time the child adored her and began to eat. But she did become very spoilt, putting out her arms every time she saw anybody and expecting to be picked up and cuddled! We got her into reasonably good condition and sent her home. She was walking by then, probably for the first time in her life, and the parents continued to bring her to the Clinic.

Another case, of which we never knew the final outcome, was that of a little girl of about ten from a poor family who presented with fairly advanced tuberculosis, certainly of the chest and almost certainly of the abdomen as well. Every treatment tried made this little thing sick. For weeks we struggled and eventually found something that she could take that would prevent her vomiting, and she really began to mend. We kept her in hospital for as long as we could, but the parents, and she as well, begged eventually for her to be allowed to go home. She was obviously fed up with hospital, and the parents lived fifteen miles away, so it was costing them a fortune to come and visit her. So with strict instructions written down in Nepali, and her tablets all carefully labelled, she was sent off home. About a fortnight later the family turned up on our doorstep with a live chicken as a present, which to our embarrassment they insisted we accept. But we drew the line at eating it, and kept it for a while as a pet until it disappeared. The girl came back for her next appointment, still improving; and then we lost sight of her. This often happens when T.B. patients start to feel better — they give up the treatment.

She was only one of hundreds of tuberculosis cases we came across in our first few months alone, and it soon became apparent that among the many problems that surrounded us this was one on which we really could make a major impact.

Less than forty years ago this disease was all too common in the British Isles. Sanatoria housed hundreds of patients, who had simply to be kept isolated from the outside world because no medicines existed to combat the disease. The wealthy flew to Switzerland, where the clear mountain air aided the possibility of recovery. The poor coughed their way to blood-stained death wracked by pain, and shrivelled to sad skeletons of skin and bone. Crowded living conditions and poor nutrition aided the spread of the disease. Then the advent of streptomycin, which kills the tuberculosis bacilli, and the introduction of the B.C.G. vaccine which provides effective protection against infection, virtually wiped tuberculosis out. Today in Britain it is comparatively rare. But many areas of the world are less fortunate, and Nepal is one of them.

Tuberculosis stalks everywhere in Nepal: in the Terai, in the foothills and in the mountains. As communication increases so the disease spreads from village to village, from community to community. Nobody can avoid contact with the droplets carrying the deadly organisms, which are borne in the air blown from the dusty streets. One infected man huddled with his family around the fire will soon infect all, children and adults alike. Pathetic skeletons crawl to the hospital gates to die within hours in the small infectious disease block. Possibly as many as three out of every hundred of population are tubercular and we felt that we had the opportunity of trying to improve this situation.

The Terai area of Kosi Zone was conveniently divided into two districts, one on either side of the single road that joined us to Dharan. Each district was further divided into areas under local Government (Panchayat) control. The number of people in each Panchayat varied considerably, and in many cases it was quite impossible to obtain a reliable population estimate. Our scheme was to visit each Panchayat systematically and to give B.C.G. to every child from one day old to fifteen years. Fortunately, to achieve effective reduction of the future incidence of tuberculosis, vaccination of 64% or more of the total number of children in an area is sufficient. Discussions were started with His Majesty's Government and the Director of the World Health Organisation in Kathmandu, and detailed plans drawn up for publicity, supplies of equipment and vaccine, and methods of reporting statistics. As early problems were overcome so more took their place, but as the weeks went by they were gradually solved and we were ready to begin.

A Panchayat would be chosen and a letter sent by the hospital Health Educator to the senior official (Pradhan Panch), advising him that a publicity visit would be made on a certain date prior to the actual day when the vaccination teams would arrive. The publicity visit was usually made by the Health Educator and one or two members of our own staff. Much depended on the local officials; for after full discussion it was their responsibility to inform all the villagers and to arrange for centres to be set up from which the vaccination teams would work.

Now we were to learn about the Terai; about its rivers and jungle, paddi fields and sugar cane, buffalo tracks and swamp; about its people and their customs; about their homes and their helplessness, worries and ambitions.

The absence of accurate maps made it necessary for our driver to make a detailed reconnaissance first, to ensure that each vaccination centre could be reached by our landrover. We soon learned to doubt local advice that a particular road was passable, after we were casually directed into a river which proved to be at least five feet deep. Sahib's car could obviously go anywhere, but even landrovers have certain limitations! We never actually turned the vehicle over in the Terai, but there was one occasion when Peter was able to stand upright on the inside of the door. The Terai is an area of great beauty and great contrast, criss-crossed by rivers and buffalo tracks. The brilliant green of the rice fields blends with the darkness of the forest. Bananas, mangoes, paw-paws and coconuts cluster round the tiny villages. Beyond, are fields of sugar cane and jute.

Birds are everywhere, from the tiny Bee-Eater to the giant Adjutant Stork. There is no country in the world which has such a variety of birdlife.

On Thurdays, early in the morning, the landrover was loaded with equipment and the vaccination team, usually including a doctor, who did his best to treat the many patients brought to the vaccination centres. Nepali and British nurses squeezed into the car, equipment was stacked into the cupboards, thermos flasks of ice were strapped into position and away we went.

If all went well we would drop a team of two at each pre-arranged centre, and the car would then be used to drive round the area collecting wayward children. The chance of actually travelling in a car produced such enthusiasm that frequently we had twenty to thirty of them packed in. This made for more problems when we became suspended on the ridges in the track and had to dig ourselves out! On one occasion a crowd of laughing villagers lifted the landrover bodily over a particularly difficult section.

There were days of frustration when local publicity was poor and few children arrived at the centre, and others when we could see hundreds of people converging on the centre from every direction.

I will never forget the day when we had to drive for nearly three hours to reach a particularly large Panchayat, which we knew to have at least 2500 children. It had a fairly large representation of ex-Gurkha soldiers and a very active Peace Corps Volunteer, Bernie. He was quiet but very well liked in the Panchayat, where he had made a great number of friends. He promised to help arrange things and as we approached the first centre, the main school in the area, we knew we were in for a busy day. Bernie and the army had done their publicity and the organisation was wonderful. The bigger children were lined up in row upon row, and behind them were the families with the younger children. The eyes of our two senior Nepali nurses, Kamala and Shanta, lit up — they revelled in their work, and were always happy if the numbers were good, but quiet if the day had not lived up to expectations. In five hours that day, 2496 children were given B.C.G. — a record we shall never beat. A very happy and tired team sang Nepali and English songs all the way back to Biratnagar.

Soon the word was getting around and Panchayat officials started to come to Biratnagar to ask for their areas to be visited. But with the monsoon not far away we knew that the tracks would become impassable and that we would have to limit ourselves to areas close to the road and to schools and factories in the local area.

Our last trip of the season was perhaps our most amusing of all. Less than two miles from Biratnagar the landrover stuck firmly in thick mud, and it looked as if it might disappear altogether if it was not moved quickly. Two enormous buffalo were enlisted to help, but all that happened was that we were all soon covered in mud, and exhausted. Fortunately we were able to find a tractor, which almost blew up before we were eventually pulled clear. Late already, we decided to abandon the car and to reach the centres on foot. Kamala and a young student nurse were a trifle surprised to find themselves bundled into a buffalo cart, and it was only when shrieks of laughter came from the other Nepali girls that we realised that we had sent off two unchaperoned girls with an unknown man. All was well however, and Kamala reappeared later in the day after giving nearly four hundred injections. Mud, dust and water had no effect on the nurses' morale, as with saris hitched up they would wade rivers and trudge through thick black mud to reach their objective. At the end of a day they would return to the hospital grey with dust, bruised and battered, tired and yet still laughing and smiling.

One Panchayat was extremely persistent in its demands for our team, but with the tracks now deep in mud and the rivers rising there was no chance of taking the car, so it was decided that Gill and I should try and get through on our two Honda motorcycles. For mile after mile we skated our way along deep ruts and through rivers. Children and parents stood open-mouthed as we weaved our way through villages. Cows and buffalo, goats and chicken stampeded into the distance pursued by their laughing owners. We reached our destination and were surrounded by a hoard of officials and inquisitive villagers. Their astonishment knew no bounds when Gill removed her crash helmet. Nobody for one moment had expected to see a girl, especially one dressed in trousers and boots. We walked for miles that day, but unhappily, although the officials were enthusiastic and helpful, the population were mostly Mardesi, a very poorly educated tribe of Indian origin, who could not, or would not, attempt to understand the reason for the injection and no amount of explanation would bring them to gather their families together. This tribal group always caused us the greatest trouble, and this day was no exception. In the gathering dusk we started for home and just as I was negotiating a particularly steep and muddy bank I heard an unladylike cry from behind me, and turned to see Gillie sitting in a sea of mud with her bike sliding down the steep bank. Uninjured but very wet she managed to get going again, by now very tired and longing for a hot drink. Two miles from home our landrover appeared, with almost our entire staff on board. They had been worried lest we had got lost or broken down, and had turned out to search for us. The 'Sergeant' produced the inevitable bottle of *raksi* and, refusing the offer of a lift, we summoned up our limited remaining energy and slowly ground our way home.

CHAPTER XV

Adapting Ourselves

These first eighteen months, when we were still getting to know each other, and at the same time learning how to work in a culture alien to our own, proved to be the most difficult we were to face. However well one gets to know someone in the comparative comfort of life in England, it is impossible to be sure of their responses to working seven thousand miles away from home in conditions totally different from anything previously experienced. In addition, our own community was a very small one, so the natural outlets for emotional tension were restricted. Barney was the best equipped for such work, in that a year working in Nigeria had prepared him.

The first thing we had to do was to try to learn to understand Nepali ways of life and ways of thought. Without such understanding we would be unable to communicate, and thus to teach them our own methods of nursing, doctoring and administration. Striving to obtain immediate perfection was of no value: improvisation and repetitive demonstration had to be our strongest allies. During this early period we had not learned to give and take among ourselves, and strong differences of opinion sprang up between team members. Minor molehills often grew into mountains. There were so many improvements that we wanted to make, that we tended to quarrel about priorities. Each person tended to become involved in his own speciality and had little time to involve himself in the difficulties of others. So it says much for the nurses that they were able so soon to make an impact in their own fields.

Rosemary set about improving the standard of the midwifery department, which dealt with a large number of deliveries although there was only a very small ward and a single 'labour room'. Because of the lack of antenatal care many of the deliveries were grossly abnormal and the death rate among both babies and mothers was very high. The tragedies which happened almost daily were accepted as routine by the Nepali staff, and improvement seemed very far away.

Rosemary started by trying to improve sterile techniques. She concentrated on simple things: seeing that equipment was always available, that sterile gloves were always at hand, and a small table was arranged in the corner on which newly born infants could lie as the doctor or the nurse sucked the mucus out of their lungs. She got on with her own Nepali nurses well and she made them understand how necessary it was for changes to be made. And when a year or so later the new Department was built, although by then she was home, it was to incorporate many of her ideas and to prove very successful.

Prue was responsible for establishing a new Children's Ward. Although it had only five beds, it accommodated the really desperately sick children who came to the Out-Patient Department and to the Children's Clinic. As in the Midwifery unit, there were tragedies — pathetic children brought in after the 'witch doctor' had failed to cure their raging dysentery, with skin so dry that it could be folded, lustreless eyes sunk into shrivelled skulls and limbs like matchsticks. These often arrived too late for successful treatment.

However, there were also the other occasions when the seemingly impossible happened and the million-to-one chance became a reality. Kanchi, for instance, was eight days old when she was brought to the hospital with tetanus. At home in the dirty mud hut the umbilical cord had been cut with a filthy *kukri* and the infection had entered the bloodstream, producing spasms when the tiny body arched almost double and the face contracted into a dreadful grimace. There seemed no hope, the child must die of exhaustion within hours. But heavy sedation reduced the spasms, and the nurses put everything they had into saving Kanchi. For day after day, night after night, a nurse stayed by the bedside sucking secretions from the throat, feeding milk down a tiny gastric tube, and trying to keep the child as quiet as possible. The mother had almost no milk of her own, but Penny was feeding Andrew at this time, and she had fortunately more than enough, so the excess went to Kanchi. Slowly the spasms subsided, and strength flowed back into the frail frame. Three years later a normal healthy child attends the Children's Clinic with a very grateful mother.

Prue now left us to work in Darjeeling; and Peter had already left for Australia. This had always been his intention and although we were sad to lose him, he had done the job he had undertaken, and much more. He had seen us safely through our journey and helped establish us and make us comfortable. Anything none of the rest of us wanted to do had been handed on to Peter, and he had coped when most others would have given up in anger or disgust. Indeed, he had grown up considerably over that year, and from being an unsure and rather unhappy boy had become a purposeful, confident young man. This was not to be the last we were to see of him.

In the middle of the second year Di and Vint, Sheena and John would be returning home, but meanwhile they were to have a second stay in Dankhutta. The people in Dankhutta still talk about John's skill as a surgeon and wonder when he will return. For there are in Nepal an enormous number of deformities requiring surgery: dreadful contractures from burns, congenital hair-lips and cleft palates, and enormous thyroid glands sagging down on to shoulders and chests.

Vint and Di not only started the laboratory in Biratnagar, but were also responsible for the firsthTuberculosis Clinic in Dankhutta. Two tiny rooms in the grounds of the hospital were their only working space, but the foundations had been laid and the local people had gained the confidence to build on them themselves.

At home our Trustees were finding it difficult to recruit doctors and nurses, and the situation was becoming desperate, for we would lose the confidence of the local people and of the Government if replacement staff could not be found to carry on our plans.

Gillie had to face this period alone in Biratnagar. The theatre had improved out of all recognition and the Nepali staff really had begun to take a pride in their work, but the actual space was woefully inadequate and the temperature so high in summer that all the windows had to be opened, thus increasing the risk of wound infections. Fortunately, Gillie had managed to find another room for the paraffin autoclave, which previously had been next to the theatre, its fumes adding to the discomfort of all concerned. A technician had been trained to work the machine and sterilisation techniques were vastly improved.

Joe was operating almost every day, which put a great strain on the theatre staff, and Dr Bharat was more than pleased to hand over anaesthetics to Penny, so that he could deal with administration. Joe had to, and did, cope with everything: bullet wounds, multiple fractures, crushed chests, fractured skulls, perforated ulcers, bear bites, and Caesarian sections. He still managed to keep up a flow of banter, which helped the nurses keep a sense of humour as their gowns turned sodden in the heat. Joe was the one of the local staff we really knew best of all, and it was he who showed us that the Nepalis have the same sense of humour as we do. Double meanings and dirty jokes are enjoyed in the same way, except perhaps that Nepali nurses try hard to be inscrutable and pretend that they do not understand, although the laughter in their eyes rapidly gives them away.

Some very remarkable cases came to theatre. It has often been stated that appendicitis is little-known in countries where Western processed food is a rarity. We saw several cases, but more often than not we never found the appendix. Where it should have been there was only a hole, spilling-out faecal contents into the abdominal cavity and causing dreadful peritonitis. How these patients managed to walk for days to get to hospital, let along survive an operation, remains a mystery to all of us.

Peter Fisher came out to join the team for a year, before going up to Cambridge to start on a medical career. He was the first of many students to work with the team, and these were to be responsible for the day-to-day organisation of the Hill Drug Scheme. This involved the purchase of drugs from India, and arrangements for their distribution to the retailers in the Hill villages. It also entailed frequent tours, both to ensure that the system was working well and not being abused, and to look into possibilities for expansion.

CHAPTER XVI

Accident — and More Problems

We reached our lowest ebb on a dark and wet night in mid-July, 1969. Barney had returned to the U.K. for a few months to get married, and I had taken over the East-West Highway, so this left only Gillie, Peter Fisher and Penny in Biratnagar. David, an officer from Dharan and a frequent visitor to our house, had gone with Gillie and Peter to Darjeeling for a well-earned weekend's rest and on their return journey along the narrow Indian road from Siliguri to Purnea they were suddenly confronted by a set of headlights weaving their way wildly down the middle of the road towards them. The skill of the Gurkha driver saved them from a head-on collision: wrenching the wheel sideways and braking hard, he manoeuvred a side-impact, which resulted in extensive damage to the vehicle but less serious damage to the occupants. Nonetheless the situation was critical. The driver of the lorry fled into the darkness, as is the usual practice in such circumstances in Nepal and India because crowds gather quickly and it is not uncommon for the driver to be beaten to death before the police arrive.

The police did arrive and were extremely courteous and helpful. An armed guard was placed on the landrover to prevent it from being stripped down to the chassis during the night, and the occupants were taken to the local hospital. Gillie was the most seriously injured, with severe cuts to her face, and everyone was in a state of shock. In the tiny ill-equipped hospital everyone was made comfortable and Gillie was stitched: not even local anaesthetic was available but, numbed by the crash, she remembered little of the pain.

To add to her discomfort a fan was directed on to her, above which was perched a bird's nest, which produced a totally undesired effect!

Fortunately another vehicle was returning that night to Dharan from Darjeeling in which was someone who knew us: Bishnu Rai, a Q.A.R.A.N.C. (member of the Queen Alexandra's Royal Army Nursing Corps) from the Military hospital in Dharan. She recognised our landrover, derelict at the side of the road, but had of course no means of knowing what had happened to the occupants. The only thing she could do was to race back to inform Penny. A landrover was made available immediately by the army, to pick up Penny, batter its way back into India and find out what had happened in the crash.

Penny remembers this sixty-mile drive as a nightmare. Had anyone been killed? Or injured? And how severely? Was the car irreparable? At last they arrived at the little hospital, and found everyone alive and not too seriously hurt. The police arranged transport back to Biratnagar, but the journey was a terrible ordeal for Gillie, whose face was beginning to give her severe pain.

The next few weeks were very difficult for Penny, and she would have found it impossible to cope without the help of our friends from Dharan and Biratnagar. Not only did she have to do her work in the hospital and most of the administration, but she also became a nurse to Gillie, who was soon suffering from severe headaches, as well as double vision.

Never again were we to be in such a difficult situation. Peter Baker, our replacement doctor, and two nurses, Hilary (Hillie) Robinson and Jane Gray, were on their way out overland; and a married Barney was soon to return with Rachel (Roo).

Hillie was to take over from Gill as our Senior Nurse. She was round and very jovial, and although she had a difficult task in stepping into Gill's competent shoes — I think she found that so much had been done already that she had to look very hard for other work — she soon became involved with the Nepalese nurses, who liked her very much, as did we all.

Jane was small and slim, but so tough and wiry that she was able to do a man's job as well as, if not better than, he. She thoroughly enjoyed the outdoor life so she was allocated to the B.C.G. unit. She got through the hills at amazing speed, I think she was faster than all the men on the downhill trips, which always were the most exacting. One of the problems a lot of us found was that our knees hurt us when going downhill, for the descents were so steep that the pressure on the knees was quite considerable. But Jane was a perfect gazelle in the way she leapt down the hills, and was to be found drinking tea in the little *bhattis,* even starting on her second cup, long before we caught up with her.

Peter, Hillie and Jane came out overland, bringing a new landrover to replace one of ours that had finally given up the ghost. Peter reminded me of the British Ambassador, with his long sideboards and dignified manner, but he was soon to fit in to the work of the Trust, and it was mostly due to his efforts that the Tuberculosis Clinic in Dankhutta was to get off the ground.

The Pathology Laboratory was becoming increasingly busy and we were fortunate to find an ex-Gurkha, Amarbahadur Pradhan, as laboratory technician who had wide experience especially in the field of blood transfusion.

Blood was always desperately required in every department of the hospital: for expectant mothers, for bleeding ulcers and for surgical emergencies. A normal level of haemoglobin in the British Isles is 100% for a man and 85% for a woman. But in Nepal these figures were never approached; in fact anyone found to have a figure within the normal range was treated as something of an oddity. Poor diet is mainly responsible, but hookworm and other gut parasites take a heavy toll.

People were usually very reluctant to donate blood, an

attitude that stemmed mainly from ignorance, although religious beliefs played their part. Relatives had to be gathered together and a careful explanation given to them that if no blood was available an operation could not be undertaken. Gradually, as patients were seen to recover, this reluctance was overcome and a service established which was to save many lives. Students from the local college responded to our appeals, and as Mr Pradhan was himself studying at the college in his spare time, a donor system was set up. Over 200 students came forward. They were grouped and each given a card to carry with him. An urgent call for blood would send various members of the staff careering round the town on bicycles routing out donors, who on many occasions turned out in force to offer their help.

One dramatic case that had a happy outcome was that of an important man from a town some ten miles off, who had a suspected cancer on which we planned to operate. For this we required blood, and our donors turned out to be a man who had at one time been Prime Minister, no less, and a woman who was the first wife of a very wealthy landowner. Everybody was lined up outside the theatre, among them the ex-Prime Minister. The patient was very scared. Then Penny started to anaesthetise him while the surgeons were scrubbing up, and his heart stopped. Of all the patients for this to happen to, this was probably the worst from the point of view of the prestige of the hospital and the surgeons. We got him going again, but the operation could not be done, the risk was too great. He was sent later to Calcutta where he was given radiotherapy instead, and he recovered.

Some of our theatre cases were now very high-powered, with the advent of Dinesh Gongal, the new surgeon. He had a lot more experience than Joe Bhattacharya. In contrast to Joe's tall, rather good-looking appearance and slow Nepali attitude to letting things take their course, Dinesh was small, wiry and quick. He was somewhat short-tempered on occasions but really extremely pleasant to work with, and he took the hospital by its ears, re-organising it and insisting that his theatre cases should be given utmost priority. On one occasion he had a patient who had to have a lobe of his lung removed for T.B., and since there was no one else, Penny had to give the anaesthetic. This was way beyond her experience, so she mugged it up from the book and then, with Dinesh's instructions, managed extremely well. Similarly, an operation for a brain tumour was carried out successfully.

The Children's Clinic was expanding — in fact it was bursting at the seams and we looked forward to the day when a new building would be opened with the help of a United States Aid Programme. In the meantime the house where Di and Vint had once lived was adapted to cope with the rising tide, thus relieving the hospital Out-Patient department of some of its load.

The atmosphere of the clinic was changing in many respects. We were beginning to establish a system whereby mothers brought their children for regular check-ups, rather than only when they were ill. Many mothers treated the clinic as a place where they could display the health of their own babies to others, so creating a standard for the less fortunate to aim at. The place still resembled a rugger scrum, but the referee was not required quite so often to settle fights about who would be next to see the doctor. Healthy babies were screened by the nurses and the ill ones by the doctors. Dysentery was the most common presentation, because the mothers were often totally ignorant of hygiene. Babies would be brought in with filthy bottles filled with unboiled water. Repellent-looking dummies were stuck into mouths, and many babies had scabies and lice. Barney took great delight in hurling the bottles and dummies out of the window, while Nepali nurses carefully explained spoon-feeding and the necessity for sterilisation. In some cases no amount of explanation would have any effect, and we would have to admit the child so that we could ensure adequate nourishment for it, and enable the mother to see for herself how it should be looked after.

Young mothers of twelve or thirteen years of age were common: we would often mistake them for older sisters. They were blissfully unaware of even the most elementary rules of child-rearing, and found it very difficult to develop any sense of responsibility.

Smallpox and B.C.G. vaccinations were given to every child, and soon we were to start to give triple vaccine, (which unfortunately was in very limited supply) as protection against diphtheria, whooping cough and tetanus.

Diphtheria is rarely seen in England now, yet only thirty years ago it was common and often fatal. We saw many cases in Nepal, and it is not a pleasant sight. Grey-faced children were carried in gasping for breath, and a foetid odour hung in the air characteristic of the disease. On looking down the throat one could see the tell-tale membrane covering the back of the throat, which bleeds if one tries to remove it. The toxic substances produced by the disease course round the body, particularly affecting the heart. In severe cases tracheotomy must be performed. This involves making an incision in the throat and inserting a tube into the wind-pipe through which the child can breathe, and secretions can be sucked out to clear the lungs of fluid. This requires skilled nursing, especially as the children become extremely frightened when they find that they cannot talk. One cannot leave them for a moment lest tiny fingers try to tear the tube out, resulting in death from asphyxiation if it is not replaced immediately.

As time went by we became accepted as full members of the community. No longer did people stare at us in the streets, wondering what we were doing there. When we said to each other that we were going home, we meant that we were going to Kafle Niwas — not to the British Isles. The local people gave us every encouragement and welcomed us into their houses and we returned the hospitality.

Major Thapa and his wife Devi were the first people to make us really feel at home, going out of their way to introduce us to their friends and to teach us their way of life.

Babar was an ex-Indian Gurkha Major, and a great ally. His advice was always welcome, his wealth of information always accurate, his humour never dimmed. He had been captured by the Chinese during the fighting with India, and had many interesting stories to relate. Devi was a lover of the arts, and a woman who could never think ill of anyone. She was widely read, and would discuss politics, religion and customs as readily as cooking, clothing and etiquette. Perhaps by now she has persuaded Babar to buy a house in Dankhutta, where she yearned to live.

We were conscious that it was a special privilege to be invited to meals with Brahmin families, such as that of Kos Raj Regmi, who published the local paper, and Professor Sharma, a teacher in the nearby Morang College. It is very unusual to be invited to a Brahmin home, let alone for a meal, and even more unusual for members of the caste to come to one's own house. I am sure they found it as difficult as we did to make the original gesture, but simple etiquette such as washing one's hands before a meal and eating with one's fingers using only the right hand soon became natural to us. In their turn our friends would go to the trouble of supplying us with cutlery. In fact, we found it was far easier to eat with our fingers!

Apart from small dinner parties we tended to give a buffet-supper on the average twice a year, inviting the British families from Dharan and local Nepali friends and officials. One might have expected these to be rather staid affairs, but this was not usually the case. The girls became experts at manufacturing an extremely potent punch made from local rum, and a large tent was erected in the garden, which served as a bar. Local beer was also available and occasionally we had some of the 'real stuff', to which Joe was extremely partial. All our staff were recruited to help and were dressed in uniform of white trousers and coats, except for the Sergeant, who appeared immaculately turned out in full uniform with the inevitable *kukri* at his hip. He directed the parking of the cars and repelled any unwanted intruders. Dhan Bahadur, our cook, disappeared into the kitchen twenty-four hours before one of these events, and never failed to produce excellent food sufficient for as many as seventy guests and suited to their varying tastes.

These parties were intended as some recognition of the extraordinary hospitality offered us by the Officers and Sergeants and their wives in Dharan. The Officers'and Sergeants' Messes were thrown open to us. We were invited to swim, ride and play golf. We became house guests and were even lent houses to stay in when people were away on leave. Everyone in fact went out of his way to help us, and we were and are still very grateful.

In our small way we too held open house for anyone who wanted to call, and our verandah was frequently overrun with Corporals and Colonels, doctors and diplomats. We provided a haven in particular for anxious travellers, marooned while the Royal Nepali Airlines decided if and when they were likely to have an arrival or departure.

CHAPTER XVII

The Hills Again

Now that we had a full complement of medical staff again, plans were going ahead to extend the B.C.G. programme into the Hills, a totally different problem from the Terai.

Ganga Shresth was our retailer in Dankhutta, chosen by the local Panchayat to sell the medicines we supplied through the Hill Drug Scheme. This he did with great integrity and considerable enthusiasm. And from him we rented a small house near the hospital for our T.B. Clinic. It was situated in the main street, in an ideal position to attract customers, and had two floors, so the doctor could work upstairs and the nurse down, registering patients and collecting blood and sputum samples.

Peter was thrown in at the deep end. With no knowledge of the language he set out to evolve a system of diagnosis and treatment which would be suited to the conditions. The local Nepali doctor referred patients with suspected T.B., and posters attracted others who, if found not to have T.B., were referred in turn to him. Diagnosis depended purely on finding the bacilli in the sputum of the patient, and in positive cases a regime of daily Streptomycin injections was started, and one daily tablet of Thiazina prescribed. Streptomycin was given daily for two months, but Thiazina had to be continued for two years.

For those living locally, daily injections were no problem, for even if they failed to arrive at the Clinic, nurse or doctor could visit them at home. Patients would in any case think nothing of walking for up to two hours for their daily injection and two hours home again. But those living further afield had to be persuaded to live in the town during this initial two-month period. Some refused and had to be treated on Thiazina alone, returning fortnightly or monthly for additional supplies. Others lived with friends or in the shelter of the Temple, often fed by local people if they had no money to buy food. This regime brought about dramatic improvement in many, and the popularity of the Clinic grew. Unfortunately, as happens with many comparable conditions, patients may feel much better after as little as one week on Streptomycin. They will then not accept the fact that they are not cured, and fail to re-attend the Clinic. The disease may then break out in a much more virulent manner later on.

Contacts were traced and family-trees carefully constructed so that the net could be drawn even tighter to prevent further spread.

The day was long for nurse and doctor, for even when the Clinic was finished, notes and records had to be compiled and sputum and blood checked. They lacked the advantages we had in Biratnagar — staff, comfortable rooms and electricity to which to return in the evenings — and yet in many ways they were more fortunate than those living in the plains. The climate is more pleasant, the general atmosphere happier and the responsibility less. Many were the occasions when Penny and I longed for six months in the Hills.

The doctor and nurse lived in a house about two hundred yards from the Clinic, to which they returned for their meals. Kanchi, a young Rai girl, looked after the house and did a good deal of the cooking. This at first left a great deal to be desired, but with good tuition she rapidly improved, even if she was never to approach the standard achieved by Dhan Bahadur, or Pemba, his successor. Meat and vegetables were difficult to obtain at many times of the year but fruit was always in season.

The house also had its pets, two cats and a pig! The pig

belonged to Kanchi and had been given to her by a Peace Corps Volunteer. As a tiny piglet it became quite tame and gambolled gaily round the house and garden. At night it slept with Kanchi. No ordinary local pig, however, it was imported and soon grew to enormous proportions and since it still maintained its piglet customs it became an absolute menace, chasing Kanchi up the main street and tearing through the house like a tornado. On two occasions it was taken for a four-hour trek to be closeted with a local boar. I don't know if this has produced a result, but if it has passage through the main street of Dankhutta could prove by now to be a highly dangerous business.

Peter soon initiated a School Health programme, and lectures on Health Education, to make the local people more aware of hygiene and disease-prevention.

Jagnath Regmi was the Panchayat Development officer in Dankhutta, and it was his enthusiasm and help that made many of our achievements possible. John had operated successfully on his wife two years previously, and he did everything within his power to advance our plans and ideas. He spoke excellent English and at all times was courteous and enthusiastic. He had considerable influence on all local affairs and set himself the task of making general improvements in the social amenities of Dankhutta.

If B.C.G. coverage was to be effective in the Hills, there were several basic problems that had to be tackled. First, the entire area had to be covered on foot and, since we had little idea of the distances between the various villages, a preliminary survey was necessary, coupled with a publicity campaign advertising the future arrival of a team. The population of the district was estimated at 140,000, which meant that the team had to vaccinate nearly 40,000 children to achieve adequate coverage. This population was scattered over an area ranging in altitude from 400 to 8000 feet, and a single Panchayat could include both extremes. Barney and Roo, with close co-operation from local officials, divided the area into sections and made a preliminary time-table whereby they would cover one section, return to Dankhutta to replenish supplies of vaccine and food, then move on to the next.

While these arrangements were being made, Dankhutta and the immediate area surrounding it were to be tackled. The team decided to try out vaccination using a Dermojet, an implement similar to a water pistol. Easily carried in a pocket, able to deliver fifty doses without being refilled, and not involving sterilisation techniques, it appeared to be an ideal instrument for such terrain. It also had the added advantage that since no needle was involved, children were unafraid and flocked to see this new 'gun'. We were aware that preliminary trials in Korea had not proved successful, but we hoped that the new model would come up to expectations. Unfortunately, the trial merely confirmed that the apparatus was unreliable, in that it failed to deliver an accurate dose. It seems strange that in this age such a simple device cannot be made accurately, when it would be so valuable to protection programmes all over the world.

The trial did however provide us with a considerable amount of additional data on the incidence of tuberculosis in the area, and on the number of children who had acquired their own protection against the disease (that is by being in close contact with it and thus establishing their own immunity).

A local graduate was chosen to help with the advance publicity and was sent ahead to prepare the route, arrange vaccination centres and make quite certain that local officials would bring the families to the centres on the correct date.

Even in the dry season such a programme would be difficult, but this was started at the height of the monsoon, when tracks can become quagmires and even disappear altogether as landslides slice away the ground. Rivers rise by feet in a few hours and leeches leap from the bushes latching on to legs and arms.

These foul creatures are the size of a pin and difficult to

see as they hide on rock and mud, on bush and tree. They sway back and forward like snakes rising from a Fakir's basket, and they crawl through the eyelets in one's shoes and between the strands of socks, always heading for warmth and blood. They make tiny puncture-holes in the skin and can become bloated to twenty times their normal size before they are replete. To remove one's socks or shirt and find these vile animals attached to one is repulsive enough, but in addition they inject a substance which prevents one's blood clotting so that bleeding can continue for some hours after they are removed. Irritation may last for many days. In no circumstances must one pull them off and the best way to rid oneself of them is with a lighted cigarette, or by rubbing on salt or kerosene. Occasionally we would have patients in the hospital with leeches in their noses or ears, or even in the urethra or vagina. These had to be chased out, with the use of a salt solution, and grabbed with a pair of forceps before they could disappear again.

The B.C.G. programme was a highly exacting job, but in a few months Barney and Roo had given over 36,000 injections and had covered over a thousand miles on foot. There remained only a few isolated areas to be re-visited and the required numbers would be obtained.

I must not forget Tika. He didn't know how old he was and neither did we, but fifteen seemed to be a fair guess. He had been working for John, a Peace Corps Volunteer, doing some of his cooking and looking after his horse. When John was away our numbers were increased by one horse and Tika, and it was inevitable when John left for the States that Tika should become a member of our staff, so he became head-cook and bottle-washer to Roo and Barney. Quick to learn, he soon proved his value in other directions, for example during publicity visits or in the recording of the numbers of injections given to varying age groups. His wide grin was infectious, his good humour rarely diminished. His cooking however was quite appalling!

CHAPTER XVIII

Liaison With the Capital

We had to maintain constant liaison with Kathmandu, for there were always plans, supplies or permissions to discuss with Embassy staff, with Government Departments, W.H.O. and UNICEF representatives and a host of other officials from the various aid and charity organisations which seemed to increase in number almost daily. It was usually my job to conduct these negotiations, and it was on these visits to the capital that I got to know the city well.

I liked to wander round the old Bazaar in the late evening, when a quiet descended after the hubbub of the day, and cows lay placidly by the empty pathways. The town goes to bed early,. away from the main tourist hotels; I would walk into one of the little temples, silent now, lit by a few oil lamps, and look at the great bells and the prayer wheels.

I remember particularly the Temple of the Living Goddess. The goddess is chosen by the religious leaders when she is a young child, according to certain omens and the position of the stars at the time of her birth, and, like the Dalai Lama in Tibet, she can come from any family, rich or poor, near or far. In accordance with the legend she represents, she is married to a tree, and brought to Kathmandu, where she lives in her temple until puberty, after which her term of office ends and another child is chosen. Sometimes, passing through the old Bazaar, I would catch a glimpse of the goddess, and reflect rather sadly on her lonely fate, for when her term ends she often finds it difficult to find a husband and settle like more ordinary girls. In Nepal a woman's status depends very largely on her position in a family. In the cities she usually in any case keeps very much in the background, governed by her husband; but in the hills, where women do much of the agricultural work, they are often powerful, and take the lead in family affairs.

I often stayed with Dudley Spain, the Information Secretary in the Embassy. He was an ex-Gurkha, who had been on the Embassy staff since his retirement from the Army. There was very little he didn't know about Kathmandu, and I cannot imagine him anywhere else but in Nepal in the country that he loves and with the people who love him. How he managed to combine his work with a non-stop social life astonished me, for it was rare for him to have any time to himself. When he did it was spent in his garden, in which he took great pride and which was a blaze of colour the whole year round. 'Choopie' his Tibetan terrier and his cat 'Mandu' were his companions, fitting glove-like into the decor of his carefully planned house. I have a great deal to thank Dudley, for through him I was to get to know many people who could in one way or another make conditions easier for our team, and with whom I could discuss difficulties on an informal basis.

I am uncertain whether I spent more time waiting for my plane on Kathmandu airport or in the maze of Singha Durbar, but at least I learned to exercise the virtue of patience, an art apparently lost to most Westerners. Government offices had a nasty habit of being moved from block to block or floor to floor in Singha Durbar at a moment's notice, and what was the Ministry of Foreign Affairs in February would suddenly become the Home Office in April. Officials had the habit of doing the same, resulting in not a little confusion as one tried to obtain a trekking permit from the Ministry of Education or an import licence from the Department of Health. Dudley knew all the departments and those in charge of each, so he often saved me the embarrassment of addressing one head of department by the name of his lately departed predecessor.

But as we became more sensitive to the protocol involved, minor affairs were settled quickly and efficiently, although major problems had to wend their weary way from department to department as they do in bureaucracies everywhere.

The American Marines responsible for looking after the security of their Embassy held an 'open-house' each Friday known as T.G.I.F. (Thank God It's Friday). This provided an opportunity not only for Peace Corps Volunteers to get together over a glass of beer to discuss their ideas, but also to invite guests such as myself to join them. Thus we both gained further knowledge of the country, and of the particular problems they faced in their various villages. The Peace Corps had a small clinic in Kathmandu and their own doctor, and I enjoyed discussing with him the forms of disease the volunteers found themselves facing.

The counterpart in Nepal of the Britain Nepal Society is the Nepal Britain Society, and it has a very large number of members. Facilities are offered by the Embassy for film shows and lectures, and both are very well attended. People flock in: Nepali, the British contingent, staff from other Embassies, Americans, Israelis, Pakistanis, a great cosmopolitan collection of people. I used to meet new people here and discuss problems, for somehow it is much easier to discuss work in a social atmosphere than in a cold brown office. The Yak and Yeti Bar in the Royal Hotel was another meeting place, or in the summer the tennis tournament held in the grounds of the hotel.

Kathmandu is the hub of Nepal and every path reaches out from it like the spokes of a wheel. Many people indeed still regard Kathmandu as Nepal and tend to forget that there is another 46,000 square miles around it. But soon I was to be fortunate enough to journey along one of these spokes and to see another area of the country.

CHAPTER XIX

Into The Mountains

To walk from Kathmandu to Namche Bazar takes ten days. But in a light aircraft one can be in the heart of Sherpa country in just one hour.

On a cloudless morning in April 1970 I left the warmth of Kathmandu and was soon rising out of the valley and heading up towards the giant mountains of the Himalayas. My companions were two respiratory physiologists, Jim, an Englishman, and Søren, a Dane, and our object was to investigate whether or not the lungs of the Sherpas were better than those of people living at lower altitudes.

Ridge after ridge slipped away beneath us, the gigantic ice-face of Gauri Shankar sliced into the sky on our port side, and soon the hillsides turned from dusty brown to red as great forests of rhododendrons burst into view.

At 12,000 feet the air was cold and I wondered what it was going to be like living for a month at an altitude of over 10,000.

The tiny landing strip of Lukla floated into sight. The strip, originally built under the direction of Sir Edmund Hillary, is surrounded by great mountains on all sides, and it seemed hardly possible that we could ever land in such an area, but in no time at all we were bumping up the runway. We jumped down to be greeted by laughing Sherpa porters and their wives. In all the time we stayed in Sherpa country those round Mongoloid faces continued to beam their wide smiles. Sherpas can laugh even in misfortune.

Our porters eagerly hoisted our mound of equipment on to their backs and we set off for a nearby Sherpa house, where we found Sir Edmund Hillary with his wife and some other energetic New Zealanders packing up a multitude of stores to be transported to the hospital at Kunde, at 14,000 feet probably the highest hospital in the world.

Sherpa houses are nearly all built on the same pattern. They have stone walls, either thatched or tiled roofs, and the ground floor houses the animals and the top floor the family. The living accommodation comprises one large room, with a smaller room leading off it which is often used as the family place of worship. A large wood fire burns continuously, against the penetrating cold, and a bench runs the length of one wall, the wife of the house holding the place of honour next to the fire. A wooden table stands in front of the bench, and all around the room are hung kitchen utensils and, if the family is wealthy enough, great brass cauldrons and cooking pots. In one corner is the family bed — in this case it was an enormous four-poster covered with thick blankets and rugs. Guests sleep around the fire or anywhere else in the room they wish. As virtually no-one is turned away the floor can become quite crowded.

The New Zealanders were soon on their way, their porters laden, some with packing cases of food and medicines and some with rolls of alkathene piping which were soon to be used to pipe water to the people of Tangboche under the foot of Ama Dablam. We settled ourselves into our tents in a field a little way from the house, and sat down to await the arrival of the bulk of our own supplies, which were being portered in from Biratnagar, a fourteen-day trek away.

By three o'clock in the afternoon the sun had already lost its heat and we had muffled ourselves into sweaters and anoraks. So when the Sherpa household invited us to join them by their fire we accepted with alacrity. We eventually returned to our sleeping bags, mellowed by a considerable quantity of rice beer and filled with rice and potatoes.

The morning dawned cold and misty, but as the mist cleared and the sun rose, the icy peaks were covered with pink and the frost began to melt underfoot. As there was still no news of our equipment it was decided that Jim would remain in camp to await its arrival, while Søren and I took the opportunity of making a short trip higher into the mountains to visit the hospital in Kunde and the beautiful monastery of Tangboche.

At five o'clock the following morning we set off, threading our way up the trail by the edge of the Dudh Kosi (the milky river), closed in by mighty cliffs on either side. Since Søren sported not only a large beard but also a corresponding amount of hair, he soon acquired the name of 'Yeti' from our Sherpa porters, and as news of our arrival spread before us smiling people appeared to laugh and joke with us about the new 'Yeti'. We were lazy that day and at only three o'clock we stopped for the night.

Two hours later we were greeted by shouts and peered out into the gloom to find that the shouters were Jack and Mark. Mark Howarth was our second pre-medical student, who had recently replaced Peter Fisher in charge of the Hill Drug Scheme. They had brought in the equipment from Biratnagar, dumped it with Jim, and set off in pursuit of us at a terrific pace — Mark had immensely long legs and could walk at a pace that would put a strain on any of us. They had had a weary journey to Lukla but were intent on catching us up so that we could all go on up together.

Two hours of steady climbing the following morning brought us to a perch above the village of Namche Bazar, enclosed in a hollow, like an amphitheatre. We looked down into a cluster of grey stone houses and tiny fields, in each of which there were puppets carefully tilling the soil in time for the annual potato planting. The golden dome of a Buddhist temple thrust upwards out of the centre of the fields and miniature paths crossed each other in a wildly contorted maze.

Potatoes are now the main crop produced by the Sherpas, and their staple diet. They were probably introduced by the British as recently as 1840, when they presumably took the place of *makai* (sweet corn). Other vegetables are grown, especially corn, but all the rice must be brought up from lower-lying areas. Nearly all Sherpas eat meat but they don't like killing animals, so the yaks have developed a convenient habit of always choosing a Thursday to fall off a cliff, in time for the market on a Friday.

Descending into the village, we stopped to eat. Jack managed to consume a dozen eggs, while the rest of us indulged in a mountain of potatoes, goat meat and noodles, washed down with tea. Rancid butter and salt in one's tea is an acquired taste, but once acquired it stays with you — it is a very good drink indeed. The tiny shops yielded our small needs for the next few days, and soon we were once more steadily climbing towards Kunde.

With very few days for acclimatisation we were well aware of the altitude and progress was laboured, but the prospect of seeing Ama Dablam at the crest of the next ridge enlivened us as we picked our way slowly over grass and stone, sand and boulders. Mark, as always, was the first to reach the top. Gasping for breath we joined him and, without a word, gazed at the spectacle in front of us. In the distance to our right the face of Ama Dablam presented its jagged ice fields, the summit ridges sharply outlined against the sky. Closer to us the less well-known, but equally formidable, fields of Kantega and Tamasarka dwarfed the 14,000 foot ridge on which we stood. Snuggled into the valley below lay the villages of Kumjung and Kunde, and above them was the hospital. We sat and watched for almost an hour before the cold urged us on to seek warmth in the next Sherpa home.

The hospital was opened in 1965 and has been in the charge of a New Zealand doctor since then. It provides a service for over 3000 Sherpas in the area, and its staff have made extensive efforts to improve the general health of the community.

The following day we set off for Tangboche, along a path which at first contoured the mountain several thousand feet above the river and then plunged down to the river itself. Enormous water-driven prayer wheels churned their never-ending circles and a group of heavily-laden yaks ambled past us as we cooked our lunch. The final uphill trail to Tangboche was the most exhausting of all, and we stopped frequently to accommodate the lack of oxygen in our lungs. 14,000 feet is not very high by Himalayan standards, but, without any acclimatisation, it is quite sufficient to bring a leaden feeling to one's limbs on a steep uphill slope. As we crested the ridge, Ama Dablam came into full view. Its slopes go straight up into the sky above the monastery, providing a backdrop of incredible beauty.

The village was strangely quiet, which is unusual in these parts, so curiosity prompted us to ask why. It seemed that five Sherpas had been killed by a snowfall below the Kumbu glacier on Everest. All five were from the nearby area and their loss was reflected in the faces of all around us. In such a small community the death of five young men is a great catastrophe, and the tragedy set us thinking about the pressures that the increasing number of Himalayan expeditions must be putting on the Sherpa people. The toll of Sherpa deaths must inevitably grow greater and greater, and resistance from the families of the young men will no doubt increase too. Climbing a peak of well over 20,000 feet is never an undertaking to be entered into lightly. Yet the challenge of the Himalayas drags team after team of climbers from all over the world to attempt a goal which is probably, from the start, unattainable. And every time a band of Sherpa porters is called upon to set their lives too at risk.

From Tangboche the trail winds its way north-east towards the foot of Everest — unfortunately time did not permit us to go further so, after saying farewell to our overnight friends, we headed back to Lukla.

In Namche I took charge of a young Australian girl who had been admitted to the hospital in Kunde with severe altitude sickness. I don't believe that she really understood how ill she had been, for she continued to talk of future ventures into mountain areas in various parts of the world.

Mountain sickness can happen to anyone, and in the past many mountaineers have died from what has been called 'pneumonia'. We do not know the cause. We do know that sudden ascent to an altitude of 12,000 feet and above can produce a condition whereby kidneys do not function and lungs fill with water. Vomiting and dizziness often precede the crisis, and should act as an immediate signal to abandon any further uphill attempt until the natural process of acclimatisation can take place.

Back in Lukla we found Jim, surrounded by a heap of apparatus and already looking for likely subjects for the tests we needed to do.

Mark was persuaded to give a demonstration of what was required, and he set off towards the bottom of the airfield, breathing into a large plastic bag. We timed exactly how long he took to get from one end of the landing strip to the other, then measured the amount of air he had consumed.

The first trip was made at walking speed, the second at a run and the third with 35 lbs of boulders in a haversack on his back.

Surrounded by a huge audience of local people, Mark dashed up and down the airfield. The sight of a *Sahib* doing such a remarkable thing was too much for most people and they retired in helpless laughter. To carry a 150 lb load from A to B is reasonable, but to run around an airfield with 35 lbs of rock on one's back was lunatic beyond belief.

However, if Mark could do it, the Sherpas could too, and soon we had them lining up to join the party — as one porter said to me, 'This must be a joke. If we don't understand it, I am sorry, but can we play as well?'

For the next few days, we walked and ran up and down Lukla airfield — even the local Lama came to watch. Jim sat in a tent and measured how much oxygen everyone was consuming, and at night measured how much rice-beer Søren and I could consume.

Søren and I returned to Kathmandu. Jim departed to Kunde for another month and how we envied him!

CHAPTER XX

Domestic Life

Andrew was now fourteen months old and was being looked after by Bishnu, an *ayah* second to none. Bishnu had already had a great deal of experience of looking after babies, since she not only had three of her own, but had also acted as an *ayah* to a British Officer's family in Dharan. She came with the highest references and vastly exceeded all of them. Calm and serene she always knew when discipline was required, and Andrew was treated exactly as her own children were. There was always a crowd of children in the house, as all of our staff had large families, and Andrew never lacked for company. But although his first word was 'Mummy', his only language was Nepali, a limitation that was to persist until our return to the U.K. The Sergeant built a swing in the garden to which we attached a baby-bouncer. It also served as an additional washing line for Somlal, who continued to cope with his mountain of daily washing. We bought an electric iron, which we thought would increase his efficiency; it had been made in India, and its life was short — three weeks to be exact! Somlal returned to the flat-iron filled with hot coals, which he much preferred, although he would never admit it in case he might hurt our feelings.

The water pump was surrounded by a small concrete ledge and it was not very long before this became a natural swimming pool for Andrew and all the other children. As fast as the Sergeant filled it the kids emptied it, but with his usual energy, and with his jungle hat fronted by crossed *kukris* always perched on his head, he continued to keep it filled until the children's amusement flagged.

Andrew was very fair and we thought it likely that he would be affected by the sun and the humidity. In fact, this never worried him in the slightest, although Bishnu kept a careful eye on him and put his shirt on if the sun was particularly hot. It seems that young children, especially those born in a hot climate, adapt very quickly to their environment. The British children in Dharan too were able to stay in the sun long after their parents had been forced to retire to air-conditioning and iced-beer.

Makalu and Seamus were very good with the children, in spite of the fact that both dogs had been bred in a country where it is normal to tease and even to be cruel to animals. No doubt the point is that rabid dogs are common and children are taught either to keep well away from them, or to kick them out of sight.

The house and garden had undergone a total transformation. We had to resort to photographs to prove that the garden had been a mass of mud and building materials only eighteen months before. Flame trees, bananas and paw-paw spread themselves with gay abandon. Bougainvillea, coral-island creepers and rambling roses patterned the walls. The front lawn became a badminton court and the back produced vegetables of all varieties and at astonishing speed. We took a photograph of Makalu and Andrew sitting beside a cabbage, and it was the cabbage that was the largest of the trio. The Sergeant had only one failing as a gardener. His army training had led him to the unshakeable belief that everything had to be arranged in dead straight lines, and we would find him planting flower seedlings exactly six inches apart, measured carefully with a piece of string.

In the house, we had an office on the ground floor, opening from the front verandah, a dining room, a small bedroom and a fourth room which was used as a consulting room and on occasions as a spare bedroom. Upstairs we had a further three bedrooms, a very well-equipped medical library and a sitting room. The decor of the sitting room changed frequently, but it was always comfortable and relaxed. Mark had produced a detail map of Kosi Zone which we pinned up on one wall, to be added to as any member of the team travelled a new trail. We had plenty of light reading material, but the electricity supply varied so greatly that it was difficult to read for any length of time.

Electricity was always a problem, and we had to be careful to limit the number of appliances in use at any one time. If the electric iron or the toaster was in use, switching on the water pump would normally fuse the entire house. The main fuse was outside in the road, twenty feet up a pole, and could only be repaired by an electrician sent by the local Government Department. This could take many hours or even days, leaving us with candle light and paraffin lamps. An electric storm nearly always resulted in a power-cut. I remember one occasion when Gill had been invited to a dinner in Dharan and in one of her few spare moments she had found the time to wash and set her hair and prepare herself for a gay evening. Black clouds were driving in from the west and although we were expecting rain we were not prepared for the speed of its onset. Gill had just left us to go out to the car, when a howling wind and driving rain suddenly unleashed themselves. Within seconds rooms were awash and the stairs had become a waterfall, since the door to the roof had been left open. Penny, Jack and I were in the sitting room at the time and when the lights failed we shot out to close the shutters and the doors. Prem Bahadur Tamang was our bearer at that time, and we could hear him shouting in the darkness as he battled against the rain downstairs. He was filled with a large amount of *raksi,* so he kept leaving his fingers in the frame as he slammed the shutters, with disastrous results. We almost had things under control when through the door appeared a figure from the witches' scene in Macbeth. Gill's recently immaculate hair hung down in 'rats tails' to her shoulders, and she looked as if she had just been subjected to Somlal's treatment. Drenched to the skin she stood in the doorway laughing as we crawled around searching for torches and candles. There was but one thing to do. We opened a bottle of rum and revelled in the inner glow it produced, outwardly cooled by the freshness of the storm.

With Barney and Rachel back in Biratnagar and with increased staff, accommodation was once more a problem, so some months previously we had rented the house immediately opposite Kafle Niwas. It was known as Bidya Bhawan (Bidia Bough-an), and was owned by the wife of a District Inspector-General of Police. At last we had a certain degree of privacy — a very urgent requirement when several people are living in such close proximity. I must admit that Penny and I and Barney and Roo stood to gain most from this move. Cut off in Bidya Bhawan from the all-too-frequent telephone calls, and the many visitors who poured into Kafle Niwas demanding action and attention, we found the family life which we had missed for two years. However, we kept in touch through a baby-alarm we had been sent, which we adapted as an internal telephone.

CHAPTER XXI

Nurses

Nepal is desperately short of trained nurses and is attempting to remedy this situation by training assistant nurse-midwives in Kathmandu, and in three other centres in the Terai, including Biratnagar.

The first obstacle to be overcome has been that of recruitment, since many families look upon nursing as a menial occupation unsuitable as a career for their daughters. This is not really very surprising. Not very long ago the same situation existed in our own country — it required Florence Nightingale, in the Crimea, to make nursing respectable, and a long struggle to raise it to the status of a profession. And there are many doctors even today who fail to appreciate the professional standing of their own nurses!

The status of a nurse was already, and is still, growing in Nepal. But recruits have not only been insufficient in number, their educational level has been low. And a two-year course, including midwifery, was simply not enough to bring them up to the standard required of trained nurses. The girls would come directly from school, possibly to live away from their families for the first time. They were housed in an excellent nurses' home built in a large compound just behind the hospital, the junior nurses in dormitories, the senior in double or single rooms. But all the teaching was done by two tutors, and sometimes by only one, who found it very demanding trying to cram the mass of necessary information into the limited time available.

After three months a ceremony was held for the junior nurses who had been judged suitable to complete the course; and this was very much in the Nightingale tradition. After the National Anthem, the senior hospital nurse and an appointed Chairman made short speeches. The nurses in white saris — they of course wore ordinary uniforms on the ward — took the oath and each in turn received a lighted candle and had her new cap carefully pinned to her head. Tea and an assortment of sweetmeats followed, and sometimes demonstrations of Nepali singing and dancing.

A few of the nurses failed to complete the course, some because of inability to pass their examinations, others because they left to get married. Once they married it was very difficult to persuade the girls to remain in nursing, even though they were in fact bound to do so by Government contract. In Biratnagar alone there were five or six fully-trained married nurses who would not return, even to do the part-time work which could have made such a difference to the efficiency of the hospital.

Nepali nurses are paid very little, as indeed are the doctors, who receive a starting salary of less than £20 a month. Many doctors can supplement this by doing private practice, but some are not so fortunate and find it a hard struggle to maintain their families. Our salary of £40 a month, modest by British standards, seemed princely compared with theirs: from our £10 per week, after £3.50p was deducted for living expenses, all of us managed to save sufficient to go on holiday, either in Nepal itself, or to Darjeeling, or as far afield as Ceylon or Malaysia.

We were lucky in that nearly all our nurses found relationship with the Nepali nurses easy, and all of them were very popular. The learning of Nepali, especially for the first members, presented something of a problem, but a language course arranged in Kathmandu for us by the Peace Corps helped. Rosemary was very good about learning the language: she was one of those who would struggle on, not minding making mistakes, and this the Nepali girls loved. They laughed at her very often, but they were always helpful in correcting and teaching her. Hillie was another one like this. Gill, on the other hand, we used to tease because she carried on talking English for a long time, somehow always managing to make herself understood. But once she took the plunge, she was as fluent as everyone else.

Rosemary, Gill, Hillie, and Ann (another new arrival), all worked in the hospital. Jane did very little in the hospital because her sphere was first the T.B. Clinic, where she worked with Peter. After leaving the Clinic she went on B.C.G. Gill also worked on B.C.G. but remained indispensable at the hospital as well because of her knowledge of theatre work, so she never got to the hills to work in the T.B. Clinic, except as relief for a few days at a time. Hilary spent most of her time in the hospital, and did a bit of everything.

The most senior of the Nepali nurses, apart from Mrs Gurung the Matron, who for most of our time there was in Madras on a course, was Latta. Gill set about training her in theatre techniques and she became very efficient. She was a slightly dumpy, rather plain girl with a delightful smile, and underneath her slow manner was a great sense of humour.

In theatre with Latta was a less senior girl called Sima. She was a neat-fingered, very slim, precise girl who made an excellent theatre nurse.

On the other side of the hospital we had two staff nurses, one of whom had a short while off to have a baby. These two used to squabble a bit but they were both efficient in a Nepali fashion, which means to say that they knew their patients, carried out instructions correctly, but in the running of the ward, especially the paper work, they were utterly chaotic.

Another nurse with whom we worked very closely was Shanta. She was not very senior, an auxiliary nurse-midwife, which means that she had eighteen-months' training in nursing basics, public health and midwifery. She became leader of the Nepali nurses on the B.C.G. team and was a splendid girl. She never spilled the vaccine, never wasted any, and the speed at which she worked was incredible: she could do more vaccinations per hour than anyone else. We well remember the occasion a river had to be crossed during the post-monsoon period when the water was still high, and Shanta picked up her sari and waded across without a qualm! She was always sunny and for this reason was rather put upon by the others, but she didn't complain. She really came into her own on the occasion of the giant B.C.G. vaccination when Bernie of the Peace Corps and a group of ex-soldiers absolutely regimented an entire village for us, and 2300 vaccinations were done in a single day. Shanta excelled herself in innoculating 800 children in two hours, a record exceeding even that of the vaccination gun which we had tried earlier.

The hospital was a training centre for auxiliary nurse-midwives, and the nursing school had two tutors most of the time, trained girls who were enthusiastic but limited by their resources. They had few text books and virtually no visual aids. They worked from a set curriculum, which they would follow almost to the letter, and this made it difficult for our girls to help in the training programme. Eventually they persuaded the tutors to be more flexible, but for the first part of our time there most of the teaching done by our girls was done on the wards. After a while their help was enlisted in setting the examinations, and in the lecture rooms as well. This raised the language difficulty again, for although these girls were supposed to know English, because the doctors' instructions would be written in English, they could not follow a lecture in English. We all tried our hand at lecturing in Nepali, and found it equally difficult, but with the help of a blackboard and diagrams and various visual aids that we were given, I think we got the message across. I am convinced that we played a part in raising the standard of nursing all round.

The nurses kept a duty book in which all doctors' instructions were supposed to be written down. But when we first arrived this was a very difficult system to operate because the doctors would drop into the wards singly at any time. If the staff nurse was around, they were lucky, if the staff nurse was not there, they made do with a junior whose English — in which instructions were all to be written — would be inadequate. So many mistakes were made. We persuaded the doctors to run a formal ward round. Joe liked this because it reminded him of English ways. The idea was for all the doctors available at the time to do a round together, at set times, so that the staff nurse could make sure she was available, and things ran very much more smoothly after that. Nevertheless, these ward rounds differed vastly from those held in English hospitals. Doctors would come and go, discussions and differences of opinion would take place on the spot. The Nepalis diagnosed very much by instinct, and they were very frequently correct, but this made it difficult for the British to follow, especially in the case of tropical diseases, some of the anaemias for example. Joe became very accurate, judging the level of anaemia by looking at the patient's tongue whereas we would have to refer to the pathology lab for anything like such accuracy. Another of Joe's strong points was the diagnosis of appendicitis, which is very uncommon in Nepal. We would tend to diagnose it far too frequently, and then very often if a real case did crop up we were so aware that it was uncommon that we would shy away from the diagnosis. Joe knew by some uncanny instinct when to operate and when not to do so. He also knew that it was pointless to operate, whatever the medical condition, if the patient had 'lost heart'.

CHAPTER XXII

New Departments — We Start Building

From the moment we first arrived in Biratnagar the problem of the Out-Patient department had been obvious to us all. Six days a week this department was crammed with a seething mass of humanity. It resembled a cocktail party when one had gambled on sixty percent turning up, and found oneself with one hundred percent, and a few gatecrashers for good measure. Mr Dewan, guarded by a massive semi-circular desk, registered the patients, filtering off those who required only repeat prescriptions, and those who could safely go direct to the treatment room with minor cuts and bruises. The strongest reached the doctor first, fighting their way to his door. The noise was indescribable. The dispensary had only a limited supply of medicines, but these were supplied free, and in a small way we were able to supplement the stock. The poor patients were given medicine from our own supplies, and those who could afford to pay were given prescriptions to one of the local drug stores, which were legion. Owning a drug store in Nepal can be a very profitable occupation, since patients come not only from the hospital and the local private practitioners, but also direct to the shops, where some unscrupulous pharmacists prescribe their own remedies at considerable profit to themselves and not a little danger to the patient.

For the doctors dealing with such numbers of patients little time was allowed for a history, and there was only a minimal examination. We saw that these conditions could never be improved until adequate facilities were made available.

We had had the good fortune to have been put in touch with MISEREOR, an international organisation based in Aachen. It seemed that if we could produce detailed plans and a full cost estimate, they were prepared to supply the money for a new building. This would be a tremendous step forward. No architect was available, so we provided our own, and Penny settled down to design the new building, incorporating the ideas of all the hospital staff. The ground area was 2400 square feet, and this was to provide a large waiting room and six inter-connecting rooms to be used as consulting and treatment rooms. The building was to back on to the existing block, so that it would provide additional hospital space if and when required. An inside staircase led up to a new Pathology Laboratory, and two additional rooms which one day we hoped would be utilised by E.N.T. or eye specialists. An outside staircase was provided to allow staff direct access to the laboratory without having to go through the waiting area.

Penny worked for hours on the plans, and sheet after sheet of graph paper bit the dust before she had done everything to her satisfaction. The British Engineers in Dharan were not a little surprised when she arrived with pages of drawings, and were very willing to offer their advice as to the construction.

Price was the next consideration, and we asked several contractors for quotations. The results were not encouraging: estimates were far in excess of what we had expected and we suspected that each contractor was aiming to make a vast profit with which to line his own pocket.

It happened that some months previously a man named Krishna Prasad had arrived at the house and begged me to give him a job as a driver. He had been a mechanic for several years in Dharan, he said, but after leaving there he had been unable to find other work and was desperately looking for some way of keeping his family. 'Yes: certainly he could drive a landrover,' he said. So, taking him at his word, I decided to try him out. With a grinding of gears and many apologies, we made our way out of the drive, narrowly avoiding the front gate and a couple of passing buffalo. Krishna was shaking like a leaf, knowing that his job depended on the result of the test. He drove a little better on the main road, as he pulled himself together, and I told him to turn off and to see how he fared on buffalo tracks. His speed if anything increased and within a few minutes the inevitable happened. With a grinding crash the landrover took to the air and we found ourselves suspended on a rut, with all four wheels off the ground, swaying back and forth on the differential. We looked at each other for a minute, and Krishna admitted that his only previous experience was limited to the motor transport yard in Dharan. I drove home in silence. Back at Kafle Niwas, Krishna begged me yet again to give him something to do, and somehow I felt that I couldn't refuse him. Our crashed landrover was standing in the garage, the roof buckled, the doors caved-in, the wings crushed, destined for the scrap heap. I asked Krishna if he could repair it, and at the thought of some employment he almost burst into tears. At no time was the question of payment mentioned, but the next morning Krishna was there at seven o'clock, working like a beaver on the car. He not only made an excellent job of repairing it but soon proved himself capable of doing almost anything. I wondered if he could possibly prove capable of building the new department, and without hesitation he said that he could.

We worked out a cost estimate for all the items necessary to complete the construction; bricks and cement, wood and steel, paint and pipes. Including the cost of labour, our estimate was half that of the lowest contractor. The plans and costing were accepted by MISEREOR, and the new Out-Patients was born. Nearly all the materials could be purchased locally, and because it was for the hospital many suppliers allowed us a discount. The steel bars had to be purchased in India, though, so we had to resume our running battle with the Customs. The labourers were paid on a daily basis and Krishna came to me each Friday with his accounts, which were always scrupulously accurate. We had every opportunity to incorporate new ideas into the design of the building as we went along, and everyone took an interest in improving the scheme. All the floors were laid on a slight incline so that they could easily be washed down. Doors and windows were absolutely plain to eliminate areas where dust might gather. Doctors' rooms were large and all rooms had intercommunicating doors to allow easy access to other staff or to facilitate examination of patients. Since most of the patients could not read, a colour-code was designed so that patients would know to which room they had to go. As the building progressed the carpenters bent to their task of producing windows and doors and then furnishings for each room. Desks and tables, chairs and benches grew from a pile of timber, as hammer and chisel flashed in the sun.

Help and advice was ever at hand and Meen Raut, a close friend and an excellent electrical engineer, provided his knowledge to ensure that all circuits and wiring were correctly installed. Meen had spent two years in America and on his posting to Biratnagar he came to live next door to Kafle Niwas. He had a great sense of humour and was soon able to joke with us about the standard of the electrical supply which it was his unenviable problem to improve. The rapidity of the growth of the town had already far outstripped the power he could produce from two 12,000-kilowatt generators; the general wiring system was inadequate, and many individual household circuits were death traps. Fortunately, Meen Raut is a man of spirit and determination.

Krishna Prasad was never short of ideas and was so conscientious that he took up residence in the new building to make quite sure that no materials disappeared mysteriously in the middle of the night. As the building shot upwards, so did his enthusiasm. His private ambition was to build a steeple crowned by a weathercock.

Whenever a roof is completed on a building it is the custom to hold a party, and if the building happens to have two floors there is an excuse for two such affairs. All the workmen are invited and *raksi* flows freely, coupled with enormous quantities of curry and rice. I was never able to establish a reason for these parties and wondered if they were a way of thanking the powers that be that the entire structure had not collapsed under the strain.

By the time the building was complete Penny was so proud of her architectural achievement that she set about designing her 'dream' house, but I'm quite certain that it will cost more than the Out-Patients, which was built for less than £5000.

Another architect was in our midst. Barney was busily designing an X-ray Unit for Dankhutta. With the Tuberculosis Clinic fully established the need for such a clinic was obvious, and it would also provide the local hospital with an additional diagnostic facility. The project was greeted with great enthusiasm by Panchayat officials and villagers alike. And Jagnath Regmi was yet again to the fore with his advice and took a great deal of interest in the scheme.

Barney's problems were vastly different from Penny's. He had to design a building utilising only local materials, because the cost of employing porters to carry in tons of cement and steel from the roadhead in Dharan would be prohibitive; and, most difficult of all, he had to find a suitable piece of land, even approximately flat, near the centre of the village.This last problem was settled by the local people themselves. A businessman purchased a site midway between the T.B. Clinic and the hospital, and presented it for use as an X-ray Centre. Such local participation was a tribute to the many people, both Nepali and British, who had worked to improve the health of this community.

Even though local material was used, porters had to be employed to carry up certain essential supplies. Once more I was struck by the hardiness and patience of these men. I wonder how many people in Britain would be able, let alone willing, to carry over a hundred pounds up and down Great Gable twice, for seventy-five pence?

Just above Dankhutta a hydro-electric scheme was under way, which now supplies electricity to the town and the surrounding area. This involved not only harnessing the water by building a dam, but also the seemingly impossible task of bringing up several hundred pipes, each weighing over half a ton. Nothing defeats the ingenuity of the Nepalis, and we watched in sheer amazement as they built bamboo cradles around the pipes, and twelve men, six a side, lifted this enormous weight in unison and set off like a giant caterpillar up the hill side. Every man had to be approximately the same height and to move at the same pace as all the others.

The hillmen have a particular gait, somewhere between a fast walk and a trot, and they can maintain this for considerable distances without apparent effort. When stopping for a rest the leader of the group lets out his breath through his teeth, producing a whistling sound halfway between a true whistle and a sneeze, which acts as a signal for the party to come to a halt.

Dankhutta was always full of surprises, but even Barney was slightly taken aback to find a landrover sitting quietly in a corner of the town. At some time in the past this must have been carried in piece by piece, and then assembled. Why this had been done has remained a mystery: perhaps some supreme optimist had anticipated using the vehicle as a taxi whenever the road should eventually be cut through from Dharan. But although plans have been made for such a road, it cannot be built without massive financial aid from abroad, which has so far not been forthcoming. Not only will the road have to be carved out of miles of mountain, but it will also have to cross the mighty Tamar river, requiring a bridge which will take years to build. Only an access track has actually been started, both upwards from Dharan and downwards from Dankhutta, the latter as a result of the late King Mahendra's 'Back to the Village'

Campaign, under which all white-collar workers, including the Cabinet and the Prime Minister, must spend a minimum of one week in their home village every year, taking part actively in some construction work of permanent value to the area.

The road will, if built, bring prosperity to a wide area of Eastern Nepal, for it is a highly fertile land and ideally suited for growing many kinds of fruit. Oranges and grapefruit already abound; apples and peaches have been proved to be equally successful. One day these hills may be responsible for producing a major export.

CHAPTER XXIII

Noel's Visit

As more and more of our plans came into operation, day-to-day administration became increasingly difficult. It was a constant battle to keep up with accounts and to maintain the flow of reports required by our sponsors. And in addition to the major commitments there was always a mass of minor points to be covered, ranging from staff pay to new wicks for the refrigerators. Seeds were required for the garden; the water heater had blown up; someone had stolen the bananas; the cat was missing; all these served to raise frustration levels and shorten tempers.

Internal communication was a small problem, external an absolute headache. It was possible for the team in Dankhutta to telephone Kafle Niwas, but the call often proved no better than a shouting match, with one person completely deafened and the other unable to hear a word. Urgent requests were sent up and down by runners, but at best this would take no less than forty-eight hours. It was also theoretically possible to telephone Kathmandu during a half-hour in the morning, and we did manage to get through to the exchange on one occasion. This was considered a major triumph. Alternative ways were by telegram, by air document, or by hand, the last being the only reliable method.

Constant liaison with our Trustees at home was essential, but one had to allow up to six weeks for a reply to an air-mail letter. Whether they were posted in India or Nepal, documents ran a high risk of being lost altogether, and eventually we sent every letter in duplicate to try to ensure that one copy reached its destination. Telegrams or cables could be sent only from India and consistently failed to arrive. Nor were the Indians always to blame. My father almost had a further coronary when, having expected for some time to hear of Andrew's arrival, he received our telegram in an envelope sent through the normal post by our own telegraph system!

After three years the intricacies of the banking system still remained a mystery. Whatever method we used to transfer money from the United Kingdom, the result was always total confusion; it never seemed to come direct to Biratnagar. It appeared either in Kathmandu or in some even more remote place, and mountains of paper work were always necessary before it could be transferred to our current account. Withdrawing cash from the current account, on the other hand, was a thoroughly social affair. Once one had presented one's cheque to the manager, one took up residence for anything up to two hours, supplied with the morning paper and cigarettes until the cash arrived. It came as no surprise when I went to our bank one day to find that without warning it had been moved to another site!

Nearly all policy decisions were made by the team themselves, but if it became clear that opinions were closely divided we referred the question to the Trustees for a final decision. This method was anything but ideal since it was seldom feasible to explain the detailed arguments, which required considerable knowledge of local conditions; and only one of our Trustees had lived in Nepal and could understand how seemingly minor difficulties could escalate into matters of the greatest importance. So it was decided that it would be to everyone's advantage if one of the Trustees could fly out to Nepal, not only in order to try to clear up existing problems, but also to be able to return home and provide the other Trustees with a clearer picture of our future requirements.

In June 1970 accordingly, Noel Leigh Taylor, the Chairman of our Trustees, came out to stay with the team for two weeks, bringing with him Judith Croft, who was to increase our nursing staff to a total of five. This was to be a family reunion for Noel, who apart from being the Chairman, was also Penny's father.

As was not unusual, all our plans went astray. The B.C.G. programme was arranged locally so that the only serviceable landrover could be available to collect Judith and Noel as soon as we had news of the impending arrival of the plane. But perverse as ever, the aircraft arrived early and it was only thanks to Dr Bharat that anyone was available to act as a welcoming party. When he heard of our predicament, he immediately provided his own vehicle and Gillie took the wheel of a car for the first time since her crash.

It was Noel's second visit to the East: he had been in Singapore before, though in a very 'British' setting. He is a very precise person with a great instinct for diplomacy, and he allowed neither the strangeness of his surroundings nor the complexity of our problems to dismay him. What he did show was joy at seeing his family and obvious delight at meeting his grandson for the first time; but he was also careful to share his time among all the members of the team. He did not visit Dankhutta — there was not time, and it was the monsoon season in any case — but he spent hours talking, listening and familiarising himself with what we were doing. The team were immensely pleased to see him. They had all felt the lack of effective contact with the Trustees caused by the long delays in the post. And in any case, letters can seldom convey all that one means, and misunderstandings did occur. Tremendous discussion took place throughout his visit; and whether it was because of Noel's presence alone, or because of his calm personality, these discussions suddenly became very orderly and heated disagreements reduced themselves miraculously to reasoned debate.

On his journey home through Kathmandu Noel was introduced to people of note by the Ambassador, who was extremely helpful and hospitable, and there is no doubt that during his short visit he was able to form a very fair picture of our situation and our problems.

But it was not until we eventually returned home ourselves that we came to realise just how much work was involved for those in England, to keep the team going in Nepal.

CHAPTER XXIV

Royal Visit

Our friend Dr Bharat was promoted to Director General of Health, and this meant that he would soon be leaving Biratnagar, where he had done so much, to take up an unenviable job behind a desk in Kathmandu. We had got to know him very well, after our rather ignominious beginning, and knew how much Biratnagar was his home and Kosi Zonal Hospital his hospital. He had been instrumental in the building of the hospital, had watched over its slow development, and earned such respect from the local people that he had always been able to persuade them to provide money for improvements. He was indeed never satisfied with what he had already achieved, and from Kathmandu he continued to try to realise his ambition of making his hospital the best in the country.

Rumours that His Majesty the King was soon to come to Biratnagar to open the new maternity unit caused considerable stir, followed by scenes of activity rarely seen in the town. The hospital, its walls dripping with whitewash, seethed with Government officials and policemen. Archways of welcome straddled the streets, garlanded with flowers and flags. Strict security regulations insisted that only hospital staff and those responsible for the building of the unit were allowed inside the hospital compound, but the streets outside were lined with thousands of excited people who cheered wildly as His Majesty drove through the town.

At the hospital there were introductions and speeches, the King toured the new unit, and then to the surprise of his security staff requested that he should also be shown round the hospital. Then, with a roar and a cloud of dust, the convoy of cars scorched through the hospital gates and he was gone.

This quality of intimacy was perhaps what I found most impressive in the Nepal royal family. King Mahendra had lived through a period of Nepalese history which had seen the country's re-birth as a new nation; and he had spent his life striving for improvement and advance against odds that might have defeated a lesser man. For Nepal, as a small nation with no power in the world, can exist only as a buffer-state. It must thus court aid from every country, owe allegiance to none. The diplomatic problems involved in such a stance are considerable. And the continuity represented by a monarchy, especially a monarchy as active as that in Nepal, has I believe done much to provide stability to a State that depends for its very existence on a balancing act.

The member of the Royal family we knew best was Princess Princep Shah, senior patron to the Trust, who is the wife of Prince Himalaya, first brother to the King. Her many functions included the Chairmanship of the Nepal Red Cross Society, which has done so much to relieve hardship and suffering throughout the country, especially at times of natural disaster.

It is difficult perhaps for people in Europe to appreciate the scale of the disasters that are an annual occurrence in this area of the world. Cyclones and tidal waves in East Pakistan are accepted as regular occurrences and only a death toll of 10,000 or more will make news for our morning papers. Similarly, every year the monsoon takes its toll of life in Nepal. Landslides destroy homes, rivers sweep through farms and often wash away entire villages. The Red Cross makes available food and clothing, blankets and cooking utensils to the families affected by such disasters. But it may take several weeks before the true extent of any disaster is known, and during that time many may die from starvation in the steaming jungle heat, or from cold in the high mountain villages. The Princess visits many of these areas personally, and our friend Dudley well remembers the time when conditions were so appalling that journeys to the stricken areas could only be made by elephant, but even this did not deter the Princess from getting there.

The royal family have the great quality of being able to be as informal as any particular occasion permits. I remember a cocktail party when five of us were sitting cross-legged on the floor discussing mountaineering. The seats of honour, two tigers' heads, had been given to the American Ambassadress and Prince Himalaya. The King's son-in-law and the British Ambassador sat on the floor.

I also recall the afternoon of the launching in Biratnagar in 1969 of an appeal by the Red Cross, which was attended by at least two thousand local people. This appeal raised nearly £3000 in less than an hour, and Penny and I were invited to have tea with the Committee. Concentrating partly on my curry and partly on the conversation, I suddenly felt a tap on my back and a smiling face appeared over my right shoulder. 'Do you remember me?' the face said, and it was only as I produced the stock answer of 'Yes, of course, Sir,' that I realised who it was. Prince Himalaya had not been at the meeting and had slipped in virtually unnoticed.

CHAPTER XXV

Back to the Highway

In November 1970 Gillie returned home to Wales, after spending a few weeks in Malaysia with Hilary on a well-earned holiday. For two-and-a-half years she had struggled to establish a permanent working relationship for our nurses alongside the Nepali staff. She had to overcome natural suspicion and then build up a position that would command the respect of her colleagues. I know there were many occasions when she came very close to making the decision to return home, and I could not have blamed her had she done so. Not only did her nursing position require long and irregular hours of work but she also had to bear the brunt of complaints from her junior nurses, and cope with a mass of paper-work. The fact that she was one hundred percent successful in achieving all her aims was, I believe, entirely because she saw the opportunities lying ahead of us, and realised that such opportunities must be based on a sound beginning. As the months went by she could see that our work was steadily progressing away from the hospital and into the 'field' where the need was greatest. She had already worked herself out of one job, when she got the operating theatre working efficiently, fully supplied with staff and equipment.

For at least a week before she left us, invitations to parties and presents showered upon her. And on the day of her departure, when she arrived at the airport, weighed down by garlands of flowers, a surprise awaited her. The Nepali nurses with whom she had worked for so long lined the steps as a guard of honour in tribute to all she had achieved.

Our last Christmas in Nepal was rapidly approaching, and Penny and I were hoping that it would give us an opportunity to relax and spend some time together with Andrew. In fact we very nearly didn't spend Christmas together at all. It was indeed to be a time that I would prefer to be able to forget.

Since June, Cameron Bowie had been acting as our Medical Officer on the East-West Highway at Butwal. He and his wife Claire had been travelling overland to Australia, when they had agreed to spend six months in Nepal as relief for the Highway. We were delighted to have them — we would otherwise have had to spare one of our own doctors from Biratnagar. But with their ship soon to sail from Madras, they wanted to see something of Nepal before their long drive through India, and I was the only person available to take over. It took me three days to get to Butwal and for once I was grateful for the peculiarities of the Royal Airlines. With no opportunity to book ahead, I had to take 'pot-luck', and I found that the only way I could get to Bhairawa — the nearest airport to Butwal — was from Kathmandu via Gurkha and Pokhara with a quick trip to Bharatpur thrown in for good measure.

Gurkha, situated north-west of Kathmandu, is a small hill town, which not only gives its name to the soldiers we all admire, but is know as the birthplace of Prithevi Narayan Shah, the founder of Nepal. We spent several hours waiting for the plane to be loaded and I was able to see something of the countryside. The village itself is rather unimposing, dwarfed by the beauty of the surrounding mountains.

The plane we were travelling in was a D.C.3 with a difference. It was normally used for parachute training by the Nepalese army, and had two bench seats running the length of the plane. The baggage was piled down the centre and the fixed-lines running down the plane gave one the feeling that at any moment a fiery-moustached figure might appear with an armful of parachutes. Perhaps, to save all these hours of walking, one could merely state one's destination and jump out over the target area. The fact that the plane was packed with Tibetans returning to Pokhara added an air of fantasy to the whole proceedings. But it happened to be a very bumpy day and the sour odour of second-hand rice and *mumo* (buffalo meat boiled or fried in batter) tended to penetrate the dream. Tibetans don't seem to be very good air travellers!

We arrived in Pokhara in the late afternoon of the second day, and the Tibetans left us. I now found myself the only potential passenger for Bhairawa, which provided me with the excuse to stay in Pokhara and the Captain and crew of the aircraft to return to Kathmandu.

Pokhara is a place of magic. Lying to the west of Kathmandu at the surprisingly low altitude of just over 2000 feet, it provides a view of the mountains unsurpassed in Nepal. Towering out of the rather dusty valley are the faces of Machapuchare, Annapurna and Dhaulagiri, rising to a height of 26,000 feet and glaring down upon the visitor to their domain. As the plane circles the valley you can see the sprawling little town below with its cobbled streets and tiled houses. Then from the airport the road winds slowly north to the 'Shining Hospital' whose corrugated iron roofs glisten in the sun. Deep gorges carve into the valley floor and a dam guards the lake which spreads its limpid way westwards. In the middle of the lake is situated the 'Fish-Tail' — the English equivalent of Machapuchare — hotel. It can only be reached by raft but a marvellous welcome awaits the thirsty traveller from the managers, Marion and Fred Barker. Marion, an ex-air hostess, comes from Georgia, and Fred is an Anglo-Peruvian. He came to Nepal almost ten years ago, and established a camp for Tibetan refugees. He soon learned their language, to add to the Nepali and Hindi, as well as English, French, Spanish and a little German, he spoke already. At one time he sported a three-foot beard and similar length of hair, which provoked the Israeli Ambassador to address him once as 'Come down Moses'. And he was able to put his hand to almost anything. I first met him on my preliminary visit to Nepal in 1967, and when Penny and I returned in 1969 for a short holiday, there he was standing at the airport greeting us as if we had only been away for a week! At that time he was helping in the building of the Fish-Tail and living in the far less pretentious Annapurna, run by Tibetans, where you can sleep under thick blankets made from yak's wool for only 6 Rupees (25p) a night.

I spent a convivial evening with Fred at his new hotel, and the following day went on to Butwal. Butwal is a village separate from the camp close to the Indian border and almost in the foothills — but the camp itself was set in the jungle in a clearing. It was very British in spirit, which made its setting strangely incongruous. Rows of little bungalows had been built as quarters for the single men, though a few people preferred caravans, notably Lee, the catering officer. There was electricity everywhere, a big dining room with modern kitchen, and the cooks, under Lee's eagle eye, cut their vegetables on tables instead of squatting down and cutting them on the floor in their usual custom. There was a big games room where films were shown nearly every week, and at the Highwayman duty-free booze was readily available. There was a very fine little medical centre with a four-bedded air-conditioned ward, a pathology area, a tiny operating room, a clinic room, a waiting room and a verandah where most of the patients waited. There were eight medical orderlies, some of whom manned the various medical outposts stretched out along the road.

I hardly had time to get to know everyone by name before I was on my way back to Biratnagar for Christmas, and managed to complete the journey in a day which must be something of a record.

Arriving on Christmas Eve, and knowing that I had to return to Butwal yet again to await the arrival of the new Medical Officer from home, I was appalled at the thought of having to complete the annual accounts, and compile a mass of reports required in England for the New Year. And

Christmas day itself was a wretched affair. Penny was called away for an emergency anaesthetic, which kept her in the hospital until mid-afternoon, by which time I was in a vile temper as I battled with a maze of figures. On Boxing Day we completed the accounts together and then started to pack for our return to Butwal. Penny desperately needed a break and we decided to take the Renault 16, which had just been driven out overland by our new doctor-husband, nurse-wife combination, Don and Jan. We also decided to take Andrew and our new *ayah,* Thuli.

Biratnagar to Butwal by road is a roundabout distance of 574 miles, for one must first travel due south into India to Purnea, then head west to Gorakpur, and then north back into Nepal. When the East-West Highway is complete, however, this journey will be cut by half and it will be possible to do it in a day.

We checked that all our documents were in order and went to the Indian border post on the evening before our departure to make certain that we could get away early the following morning. We were assured that the post would be manned at six a.m., and that we would be cleared in the minimum of time. I even went to see the wife of the Chief Customs Officer, who was said to be seriously ill. As might have been predicted, she turned out to have mild indigestion.

The following morning we found a closed Customs post and not a sign of anyone vaguely interested in opening it. At seven a rather tired official appeared, and an hour later we were at last on our way, exasperated beyond words. Little did those officials know how close they had been to receiving permanent injury. The road to Purnea, to add to our frustration, was under repair, which involved us in frequent diversions into the countryside as the Indians have the habit of repapring both traffic lanes at the same time. We battled our way over cart tracks and through dried-up river beds and it wasn't very long before we had our first puncture. The car itself was ideal for such country cruising happily over sand, stone mud and pot-holes; but the tyres were totally unsuitable, and we had been warned by Don to expect frequent punctures. Fortunately every tiny village had at least one tyre-repair service, and we soon became adjusted to drinking large quantities of tea in a grubby shop as we waited for the inevitable nail to be extracted and the tyre repaired. I often wondered whether people were employed to make quite certain that the roads were liberally sprinkled with nails so that these businesses could maintain their flourishing trade.

Out of Purnea a main highway runs due west towards Muzzafapore, a drab and dirty town, typical of many towns in the impoverished northern Indian states of Bihar and Uttar Pradesh. We eventually found our way to the 'British Club', which desperately tries to maintain the old tradition (against impossible odds). Standing in large grounds, the enormous Victorian-style house had once been a scene of bustling activity. Officers and wives had drunk iced drinks or played tennis on the spacious lawns. Flowing dresses had adorned the ballroom and gentlemen had retired with their port and cigars to play billiards. Now the few remaining members drank their whisky reminiscing over the past; the vast ballroom was empty, and the cloth on the billiard table worn and faded. An aged retainer graciously showed us to our rooms and drinks were served on a silver tray. The rooms were vast, with high ceilings, and furnished with enormous pieces of oak and mahogany. A huge double-bed stood in the middle of the floor draped with yards of mosquito netting and cooled by the fan situated directly above.

We had been there only for about fifteen minutes when there was a sound of yet another vehicle approaching and of English voices in the courtyard. And who should walk through the door but three people we knew. They were Micky Wetherall and his wife Kay, and Desmond Wilson, who was at the time First Secretary at the British Embassy in Kathmandu. Such a coincidence was quite extraordinary since there were almost certainly no other English people within hundreds of miles! Micky had been in India and

Nepal for over thirty years, a self-taught engineer who had put his hand to almost everything including the building of roads and bridges. He and his wife lived in a caravan with an assortment of pet monkeys. There was little he didn't know about the country, and he was always willing to offer sound advice. He had been one of the few people to gain access to Nepal in the times of the Rana rule, had witnessed both the splendour of those times and the poverty, seen the regime broken and the monarchy re-established, then the country's gradual emergence from isolation.

The new arrivals caused a great deal of chaos as room space at the Club was rather limited, but Micky quickly organised an extra bed in our room for Thuli and Andrew. Thuli had dinner with us. She was terribly embarrassed, but acquitted herself marvellously in spite of the fact that she would dearly have preferred *dhal-bhat* (a wide term really meaning lentils and rice, but covering any form of curry) to our five-course meal.

After this enormous meal, the only thing to do was to go to bed. We fell asleep quickly despite the continuous hum of hundreds of man-eating mosquitoes, until we were awakened by a loud thump. It was followed by a short cry and then complete silence. We switched on the light. Thuli was fast asleep but there was no sign of Andrew. Awakening Thuli, we looked under her bed and there he was curled up in a ball fast asleep and quite unharmed.

The morning saw us again on our way to Gorakpur. We hoped to be able to reach Butwal that night, but we had three punctures, and seemed moreover to have chosen the day of the week to travel when every town and village had decided to hold either a market or a festival. Cyclists, buffalo carts, cows and a seething mass of humanity blocked every street. We were glad that Don had had the very good sense to have a 'triple-horn' fitted to the vehicle. The tone produced little or no response from anyone; the high-pitched blast produced an immediate reaction, varying from annoyance to shocked surprise, but the third variation, which sounded like a cross between a rampant ambulance and Louis Armstrong, produced astonishing results. People fell over themselves to get out of the way. Cyclists toppled from their saddles and even policemen produced a grudging smile.

It was late evening before we arrived in Gorakpur and Andrew was fast asleep in the back of the car — he had been amazingly good throughout the long and tedious journey, playing quietly for most of the time and sleeping the rest. I had stayed in Gorakpur on two previous occasions and was not looking forward to introducing Penny to one of its main hotels. It would have been condemned in England long ago. But fortunately we were the only guests and were able to choose the only room I knew to be free of bed-bugs. On an earlier visit I had been almost eaten alive by these wretched creatures, which lurk in the corners of the blankets or in tiny crevices in the woodwork. As soon as you turned out the light you could hear the army forming up for its assault. The sound of dozens of marching feet would draw closer, and as one quickly turned the light on again, the platoons of infantry were clearly visible, the front line already crawling up the bed posts. The only defence is to stand the feet of the bed in bowls of paraffin.

Gorakpur wakes early, and so did we, glad to be on the final stretch. The scenery provided a great contrast to the grey dusty land we had been driving through for the last five hundred miles. Just outside the town there is an immense fruit estate which stretches for mile after mile beside the road. Row upon row of banana trees bend under the weight of their fruit, each row stretching in a dead-straight line into the distance. Neatly trimmed irrigation ditches criss-cross the groves of coconuts and the fields of pineapples. Nowhere else in northern India had I seen such evidence of industry, nor such obvious prosperity.

In the distance the hills could be seen rising out of the plain, and we knew that the end of our journey was near. For once customs formalities were despatched quickly and efficiently, and we were back in Nepal. Our timing was perfect for we met Cameron and Claire just arriving at the border on their way into India. Cameron brought me up to date with the problems at Butwal, while Claire produced a cup of coffee for us all, on the petrol stove fitted into the back of their landrover. We relaxed a little as we drove the final thirty miles to Butwal, trying to forget that in less than two weeks we would have to drive home again.

There were two other married couples working on the Highway, David and Pauline and Dave and Mavis, and we were all fortunate to have houses to ourselves set apart from the main quarters. The presence of married couples on such a project was a subject of some controversy, I knew. But I was astonished when doubt was expressed about Andrew's presence — it was argued that he would remind people too much of their own families and might create jealousy. But as it turned out it was the married family men who spent the most time in our house playing with Andrew, who would be happily perched for hours on the enormous shoulders of Wally, the works foreman, while he directed the work on concrete mixers, stone crushers and band-saws.

Two miles north from the camp was the Butwal Technical Institute. This was a project, staffed for the most part by Germans, that had been established to teach young Nepalis carpentry and engineering. But the Institute had also embarked on a very ambitious scheme to supply electricity to the surrounding area. North of the Institute a recently-built road carved its way north through a massive gorge to Tansen and Pokhara. To build a dam in this gorge was out of the question, so the German engineers decided to divert the river through a succession of tunnels, allowing it at intervals to drop through vertical shafts, so that the resultant head of water would produce the energy to drive the turbines. They overcame obstacle after obstacle as they tunnelled their way through yards of solid rock, always aware of the danger of being trapped by a rock fall or a freak storm. Ingrid and Gerald and Angela and Walter were frequent visitors to the Highway, and in return many of the British ex-patriates spent happy evenings in their homes. Ingrid and Gerald had been in Nepal for five years and their two lively daughters spoke three languages fluently — German, English and Nepali — switching from one to the other without any hesitation.

The Base-camp had changed very little in the year I had been away, although there was a noticeable improvement in the general morale of the ex-patriate staff, most of whom were quite new to me. Lee still reigned supreme over the catering department, threatening to resign only about once a month, which was a distinct improvement on his past performance; and it was a great pleasure to see Reg, the surveyor, whose tuneless singing had amused me on my last visit, returning for a second tour. The road was really beginning to take shape and the access track had been cut through to the far side of the hill section.

This hill section could be negotiated quite easily in a short wheel-based landrover, but for the ambulance it was a different problem. Nearside vision was considerably reduced by the lack of rear windows and the position of the spare wheel on the bonnet, so the driver tended to allow more space than was necessary and thus to draw dangerously close to the precipitate drop on his own side. On our first excursion over this section my hand was permanently on the door handle, as I expected us to be launched into space at any moment; and on the way back I stopped to look at our tyre marks. In several places only half the tread was visible, and sections of the edge had simply slipped away into the abyss below.

There were now four semi-permanent advance camps, and a further brick-built camp was nearly finished at the base of the hill section. The surveyors were in a tented camp on the far side of the hill. U.K. engineers and Nepali staff lived out during the week, returning only at weekends for the Saturday night 'thrash'. At each forward camp we had a Gurkha medical orderly and an assistant, who maintained general hygiene in the camp and dealt with water supplies — water was always a problem and some camps still had to be supplied by bowsers, if drilling had proved unproductive. The communications system was greatly improved, each camp being supplied with a radio-telephone, and we also carried a radio-set in the ambulance, considerably reducing the time taken to get to any emergency. The orderlies were on the whole excellent, especially Bhoj Bahadur Gurung, who now wielded a stethoscope with great clinical acumen, and Bhakat Bahadur who in his very quiet way had acquired a great deal of confidence.

One evening I was surprised to see a U.K. engineer returning to camp with stitches just above his lip. He told me he had gone to the medical post looking for me, when he found himself flat on his back on an examination couch in less than five seconds and with three stitches in his face before he had a chance to say anything.

Serious accidents were comparatively rare, which was surprising considering the chances that were taken by some of the workers. I remember one morning when Wally reached the stone crusher to find to his horror that several large stones were wedged sideways in the jaws. The machine was still working, and two Nepalis were jumping up and down on it in an effort to release the boulders! Two enormous arms shot out and picked them out of the crusher like two feathers. We tried to impress on them that they would now be part of the road surface if Wally had not made such a timely arrival, but even this forthright information failed to remove the wide grins from their faces.

On another occasion a Gurkha bulldozer driver was ordered to clear a particularly steep bank, but instead of attacking it from the side he made a direct frontal assault. Even a bulldozer has its limits and at an angle of sixty degrees it gently tipped over backwards. The driver very neatly leapt from his seat, landed on his feet, returned to the dozer which had by now turned a full somersault, and renewed his attack yet again. I managed to persuade him that he might save time if he made a lateral approach. His nearness to death had not the slightest effect on him.

Early in January, expecting Ian, a British G.P. who was taking three months off to take over as our new medical officer, to arrive to replace me at any moment, we started to make preparations for the return journey. The Renault needed servicing and it was arranged that an Anglo-Indian mechanic should do this in his spare time. He completed the overhaul and returned the car to the garage, but unfortunately kept the key. That night the car was missing from the garage and it turned out that he had taken it out for a test-run: two hours later we found what was left of the Renault upside down in a ditch on the road to Bhairawa. It was a miracle that no-one was killed. There was a small consolation for us in the fact that there was now no possibility of having to return by road. Fortunately a British Sergeant and a Gurkha Major were about to return to Dharan by train and offered to accompany Penny, Thuli and Andrew, leaving me to return later by air.

Ian had heard about the Trust, thought that he would like to see something of Nepal, and decided that in any case it was high time he had a change from his practice in North Wales. Now, with little time for hand-over, he found himself thrown in at the deep end. Two cases of possible smallpox had prompted us to start a mass vaccination campaign in conjunction with the Public Health nurses from the local Nepali hospital. Both cases were in fact confirmed as chickenpox; but the exercise nevertheless gained us a great deal of experience as well as proving that such a campaign was very necessary. Many of the workmen came from India, and we found that over ten percent of them had never received vaccination in their lives and that another twenty percent had not had their required booster dose during the past three years. A single case could have produced a major epidemic and brought all work on the road to an immediate stop, possibly for months.

I left Ian with a mass of facts and figures to digest, but I was confident that Bhoj was quite able to deal with any administrative problems that might arise, so for the umpteenth time delivered myself over to the tender mercies of the Royal Nepalese Air Lines.

CHAPTER XXVI

Holiday

Barney and Roo had just finished mopping-up a few isolated areas in Dankhutta district that had not been covered by B.C.G., and were now on their way down to Biratnagar to give Penny and me a chance to go on holiday together. Some months previously we had decided we would like to see Darjeeling, and had managed to persuade the Indian authorities in Delhi to give us a permit for Gantok. We had intended to take Thuli and Andrew and to use the Renault, but the crash in Butwal sabotaged that plan, and after considerable discussion we decided to go walking in the hills. Pemba eagerly agreed to come with us, and to arrange the porters we would require to carry all our equipment. Andrew was now two years old, and still obviously too small to walk any distance, so he was to be carried in a *dhoko* (basket) in the same way as Nepali children. A very successful method this was to prove.

In order to be entirely independent we decided to take tents and virtually everything else we would need for our comfort. The mound of equipment grew and grew and as Hilary remarked, 'we might have been attempting the south face of Makalu rather than going on a two-week lazy holiday'. Food is always difficult to obtain in the mountains and we took over sixty pounds with us, including food for our porters. Some peculiar variation of Parkinson's law takes over at this point: the more porters you take the more food you need to carry, and the more food, the more porters you require. So it is best to decide on the maximum number of porters and throw things out if the loads prove to be excessive. Apart from Pemba we took three other porters, one of whom was an enormous Bhotia, named Jit Bahadur, who cruised along with fifty pounds of food on his back and Andrew sitting on the top. But it took only twenty-four hours to find out that the other two men had never worked as porters before and were unable to keep up with the rest of us, even though we were moving fairly slowly. We learned later that they had hardly ever been outside their village and had never seen the 'snows' in their lives. Mailo (the second son of the family) was twenty, and Burho (old-man) was thirty-five and very slow indeed. As we were not in any hurry, we just adapted our pace to theirs, although the delays were occasionally frustrating when we had to wait for much of the equipment to arrive before we could establish our camp in the evening. Jit Bahadur and Andrew became great friends and very soon Andrew was joining him in singing Bhotia songs as they swung gaily along the trail.

Andrew, in fact, caused quite a sensation. Many of the villages we passed through had never seen a European child. Fewer still had seen one who spoke only Nepali. He was given so many oranges that we had almost to hire another porter to carry them, and Jit Bahadur endured quantities of juice poured down his neck for most of the journey. The constant swaying of the *dhoko* sent Andrew off to sleep when he was tired, and whenever Jit Bahadur's singing lacked accompaniment we knew that this was what had happened.

We dropped in for two days to see the team in Dankhutta and then set off for Hile and the very beautiful countryside to the north. Half an hour's walk away from the village the country resembles the Yorkshire moors, rolling away treeless for mile upon mile. Mountain streams tinkle their way down the gullies and the water is crystal-clear and ice-cold. The only problem was to find wood for the fire; but a couple of miles of foraging presented no difficulties to Jit Bahadur, who set off at a terrific pace with an empty *dhoko.* It was at this point that I found myself carrying his *dhoko,* the one containing the tinned food, and even without Andrew perched on the top it was so heavy that it was all I could do to carry it two hundred yards without breaking my neck. This experience gave me even greater respect for these remarkably tough people.

That morning we had stopped in Hile at the house of an American friend who was working for the Peace Corps and helping with agricultural improvement in the area. He had as his guests the wife and daughter of the Peace Corps Director in Kathmandu, and we invited them all to come and have dinner with us. This didn't seem a very strange idea at the time, but in retrospect I suppose that in any other country than Nepal it would come as a surprise to be invited to walk for an hour to sit in the middle of a moor to have dinner, and then walk home again. But they were pleased to accept our invitation and with the rather vague instruction that they would find us roughly an hour away in a north-easterly direction, we departed to make camp. Pemba soon had the site in order, and we all returned to Hile to buy food for the evening.

It happened to be market day and Hile was transformed from a rather sleepy town into a hive of activity. Market day (the weekly *hat,* pronounced '*hart*'), is an occasion when everyone from miles around comes to the village to buy and sell. Frequently a buffalo will be killed and occasionally a pig. The main, and only, street in the town is filled with smiling faces, and the Tibetan tongue mingles with the numerous hill dialects of the eastern tribes of Nepal. The tiny tea-shops do a roaring trade, mostly in *raksi* and rice-beer. Bargaining does take place, but it is unusual among these people: a fair price is offered and you can decide either that you wish to pay it or not. No offence is taken if you decline. Eventually, Pemba emerged from the seething crowd with enough food to feed an army, and we all made our way back to his outdoor kitchen, where we found Jit Bahadur relaxing beside an enormous mound of wood.

As the evening drew in the temperature dropped and we added more logs to the fire. Pemba scurried about with pots and pans, never grumbling for a moment at being asked to produce dinner for ten in the middle of nowhere. Then in the distance we heard the sounds of voices raised in uncertain chorus 'Where the Hell are they?' Waving a torch I went to greet them, and soon we were all huddled round the blazing fire and equipped with large glasses of *raksi*. Pemba's curry was excellent: so was the company. Then, as the night closed in, we were provided with one of the most spectacular sights I have ever seen. To the north the mountains seemed almost to come alive as the moon rose above the clouds in the valleys below. Our American friends never knew how long it took them to return home, for they, like us, were transported by the tremendous majesty of the ice giants.

The following morning found us up at the crack of dawn. We dragged Mailo and Burho from their beds and made them walk up to the crest of the ridge for their first-ever view of the mountains. Indeed we had to explain to them just what ice and snow were. I never knew whether they were impressed or not, but they did have something new to talk about in their village when they returned home.

We spent two days in this magical spot and then headed north-east towards the Arun river, scene of my experiences with Keith almost two years before. Through orange groves and apple trees we descended steadily to the river and the Rai village of Sun Baluwa, which hugs the banks of the Arun at its junction with the Munga Khola. The steep descent of over five thousand feet was almost too much for Burho. We arrived at our proposed camp-site at half past four, and leaving Pemba to do the donkey-work, drifted away towards the village and the inevitable supply of oranges for Andrew. His 'calls of nature', were fortunately few, but it did come as rather a surprise to us both when a very indignant young Raini girl demanded the immediate removal of his efforts from in front of her house — perhaps the Rais are the answer to the Public Health problem in Nepal!

At seven o'clock there was still no sign of Burho, and Jit Bahadur was sent in search of him. At last at eight a very tired porter staggered in and was hustled into his tent by Pemba, who restored his sagging morale with a large glass of *raksi.* I have little doubt that this was the moment when Burho decided that portering was not for him.

Our return journey beside the Arun provided us with magnificent scenery, but spectacular as that trail is, it is one I would try to avoid in the future. At first the road clings to the river and we were able to descend gradually. Then, suddenly a view opened before us that would destroy the confidence of the most intrepid of travellers: the river dived into a gorge; while four to five hundred feet up, cut into its precipitous cliffs, lay the path that we would have to take. The only people totally unaffected by this aerial prospect were Jit Bahadur and Andrew, who swung along as gaily as ever. We hugged the cliff and avoided looking down, concentrating on our feet, until the slope eased and trees afforded us some protection. Then the river started to widen and Chattra came into view.

This tiny village hums with the throb of machinery, because the mighty Kosi river has been partially tamed and a canal — the Chattra Canal — built to supply irrigation not only for much of Kosi Zone but also for a large area of the northern states of India.

From here we were to ride to Dharan. We found ourselves packed into what must be the oldest landrover in Nepal, judging by the quantity of wire and bits of string that held it together. Frequent stops were necessary to replenish a radiator which had the capacity of a very thirsty elephant, and each halt added to the number of passengers, who eventually totalled twenty-three, those who could not cram themselves inside attached to the outside like limpets. A trifle battle-weary and very dusty we arrived in Dharan to enjoy our first hot bath for two weeks. It had not been everyone's idea of a holiday. But we had thoroughly enjoyed it.

With our return to Biratnagar we realised suddenly that our time in Nepal was rapidly drawing to an end. Of the original team that had left Southend in April 1968, only Barney remained, for the members of the first team had had no contract with the Trust and were free to leave whenever they wished. We often discussed whether this was a wise decision to have made, and I still believe it was, for at that time we had no idea of where we would be working nor of the kind of conditions we might have to face. It would only have caused further difficulties if unwilling people had to be forced to complete contracts in conditions they found intolerable. By the end of 1969, however, we had a very good idea of how our work would develop, and were able to give applicants at home a fairly accurate picture of what they would be expected to do — and what problems they would have to face. We decided that no-one should be employed for less than eighteen months save in exceptional circumstances, and that we should try to find people willing to stay for two years or more.

I don't know why Penny and I had decided to stay for three years, but that arrangement did allow us the satisfaction of seeing things fully established, and of returning home knowing that we left them in the capable hands of Barney and Roo, people who would do everything possible to maintain and expand the work of the Trust.

That three years had also produced Andrew, and a corresponding increase in the mountain of belongings we had to arrange to ship home. We soon found out that getting trunks out of Calcutta was almost as difficult as getting them in, and we embarked on the never-ending pile of forms demanded by the Customs officials and our shipping agents. There seems little doubt that complete departments must exist to dream up new technicalities, involving more and more pieces of paper, to hamper the unhappy traveller. It is also most important that all documents should be officially stamped, so we had our own rubber stamp made and attacked each new document with it. There was indeed a marked improvement in the speed at which our various consignments were cleared. To save time we then invited the Nepalese Customs official to check our cases in Kafle Niwas before they were crated and officially sealed. He agreed with alacrity, which rather surprised us, and we were astonished when he arrived absolutely on time at eight o'clock in the morning. Liberally supplied with coffee and cigarettes he made himself perfectly at home, and by mid-afternoon it dawned on us that we had provided him with the perfect excuse for a day away from his hot and dirty post on the border. Once he was convinced that we had no intention of trying to smuggle vast quantities of hash or pieces of ancient temples out of Nepal, the crates were sealed and sent on their way to Calcutta.

Barney and I spent many hours discussing plans for the future and going through our filing system, which now filled an entire wall in the library. It was obvious that when he and Roo returned we would urgently require a Secretary/Administrator, so that the doctors and nurses could be free to do the job for which they were qualified. It was also apparent that the leader of the Trust should be based in Biratnagar, maintaining close contact with the hospital and with the many visitors from Kathmandu.

As the days went by I accumulated a massive list of decisions to be made by the Trustees as soon as we were home.

We spent several days either throwing out or giving away everything that wasn't an absolute necessity, and another week buying presents to return us to the status quo. It seemed highly unlikely that we would ever manage to keep within our baggage allowance, and everything was made much more difficult because we had to provide for a drop in temperature of nearly sixty degrees over the forthcoming journey.

The last week was spent in a whirl of parties, and up to

the very last minute we found it difficult to believe that we were really going. This country had been our home for three years, and had become part of ourselves.

Even when we were at last seated in the plane, surrounded by a mass of presents and swamped with flowers, the thought of home was far from our minds. We circled Biratnagar, looked down on its dusty streets and wondered how many years would pass before we would return.

We stayed for a few days in Kathmandu and were able to say most of our farewells at the Queen's Birthday party. Then we were finally on our way. As our plane climbed out of the Kathmandu valley we took a last look at the snows and headed for Delhi, where we were to spend a night in the Oriental luxury of Claridges Hotel. For months we had promised ourselves an evening of relaxation free to enjoy exactly what we wanted with no expense spared. With Andrew asleep and the room-boys drawing our baths, we lay back in the velvet chairs sipping ice-cold dry martinis. The menu yielded smoked salmon, avocado pears with prawns, and duck in orange sauce washed down with some excellent claret, then coffee and Cointreau. A real 'restaurant' meal, with all the trimmings, was something we'd missed for a long time, and we began to look forward to our return to Europe.

Exceptionally clear skies allowed us to trace a great deal of our previous overland route from the air. Within ten hours we crossed the deserts and mountains of Afghanistan, Iran and Turkey before turning across the Bosphorus and the Greek Islands to Athens. From Athens we crossed the Adriatic to Rome, all the time fighting a losing battle with the sun. We passed over the Alps, glowing pink in the evening light, and through thick cloud descended to Frankfurt. But late at night, having been in the air for most of the day, we found ourselves out of sympathy with the abruptness of this city. Unsmiling faces moved everywhere at high speed and our hotel room was like a prison cell devoid of anything personal except the number on the door.

A request for food to be served in our room was met with the cold information that we must eat in the dining room. The fact that we had a child to consider was not even taken into account, and it was only after I had worked myself into a fury and extracted the manager from his evening's beer-drinking that we were given what we wanted.

Not until we had crossed the English Channel and entered the circle of traffic above a rainy London Airport did we begin to conjure up pictures of our families waiting below to welcome us home.

CHAPTER XXVII

Home

We drove in cavalcade back to Farnham through a dense snowstorm. It seemed strange that the only snow we had seen during the last three years had been thousands of feet above us, capping the giants of the Himalayas — only once in the last ten years has snow fallen in Kathmandu. Andrew was fascinated and rushed round the garden trying to catch the flakes, with a puzzled look on his face as they melted in his hands.

During the next few weeks we tried to combine family reunions with frequent discussions of Trust policies, and visits to dozens of sponsors. It was only now that we realised just how much work was entailed in keeping our team in Nepal. All our Trustees were working in full-time exacting professions and yet they had somehow managed to cope with all the demands and complaints which flowed back from the mission.

In Nepal we would discuss replacements for the team and cheerfully write a letter home stating that we required x nurses in April and y doctors in May, and then sit back and wait for the conjurors in U.K. to pull them out of a hat. Little did we realise that Douglas would have to sift through a mass of previous applications and then possibly still have to advertise for the special candidate we required. As the years went by a single advertisement would bring as many as fifty applicants, who then had to be short-listed and interviewed. When the decision was made and an applicant finally accepted, contracts had to be prepared, visas obtained, dozens of queries answered, letters of introduction supplied and tickets booked. Parents would telephone Trustees at any hour of the day or night for assurance that their daughter was not being sent out to a harem in Iran, or a strip club in Tangier. Parcels of clothes and other goodies would arrive on Trustees' doormats with urgent requests to deliver them to Nepal.

The distribution of the Annual report was a full-time job in itself. Our rather scruffy reports had to be edited and compiled into a readable form. Photographs had to be gleaned from ex-members of the team, and printers bullied into producing a thousand copies at a reasonable price. Every Trust, Foundation and industrial company who had helped us in the past received a report, accompanied by a letter requesting renewed help. As more and more avenues of support opened up the distribution of reports grew larger and larger.

Fortunately my father had just retired, and was cajoled into taking over this expanding task. Looking forward to a quiet life in his garden he suddenly found himself surrounded by a mass of filing cabinets and index cards. In their hurry to please, many companies would send equipment and drugs directly to his address and not to the warehouse. Daily the postman would stagger up the drive with twenty thousand iron tablets, or five miles of cotton bandages. The house and garage looked as if they contained the proceeds of an extremely successful raid on a wholesale chemist.

Noel, Penny's father, had the most difficult job of all. Standing aloof as Chairman of the Trustees, he had to deal firmly yet diplomatically with the multitude of questions and requests that reached him from every direction. If the Trust was short of money, which it nearly always was, he had to find a way out of the dilemma. If someone decided to break his contract and come home early, the Chairman had to decide what proportion of his salary and fare should be paid. If a sponsor complained that he had not received a report, or a firm that they had not been paid, he had to find the time to humour them.

The remaining Trustees included an accountant, Dennis Turner, who somehow unravelled our three-monthly accounts sent from Nepal, and remained a member after he handed over his job as Treasurer to Fred Smailes: two more medical men, Douglas Robb and Donald Teare; and Charles Wylie — who had been in Nepal in the army and climbed Macchapuchare. Lord Hunt was a Patron, and also one of those who helped us from the start.

The project is now embarking on its second five years, and not only have the members of the team changed, so have the members of the Board of Trustees, as our work has expanded.

It may sound easy to comply with a request for spares for certain items of equipment. I had only been home a few weeks when I found that obtaining spares from companies in the U.K. is as difficult as trying to find a golf ball on a pebble beach. I had been asked to send out some spare valves for a petrol-stove. After a fruitless search through at least a dozen shops I telephoned the head office of the company concerned, who informed me that their spares department was in another city. Having contacted the department concerned I was passed from office to office, finally finding myself talking to someone who showed a slight interest in my request. He promised to send the valves to Nepal and I heard no more for two months, apart from receiving a bill for £1.20 (60p of which was for postage). When a letter arrived from Barney asking 'where the hell are the new valves?', I simply bought two new stoves and sent them out overland with our new landrover.

CHAPTER XXVIII

Looking Back

When we first went out to Nepal nearly seven years ago, we saw ourselves setting out to do a limited job — to take part in and help improve the work of a local hospital — and though we hoped to extend our work into the hills, and soon saw the immense need for work in preventive medicine throughout the country, we knew that our long-term success would depend upon building a solid base. And success here meant working ourselves out of the job we were taking on.

In concrete terms, we can now see what we have achieved. There is a Pathology Laboratory in Biratnagar Hospital, a Children's Ward, a new and efficient Out-Patients' Department, all staffed by Nepali nurses and technicians whom we helped to train. In Dankhutta there is a new X-ray unit and a T.B. Clinic, and there are two more T.B. clinics in Chainpur and Ilam. Nearly half a million B.C.G. vaccinations have been given, protecting the entire Kosi zone and most of Mechi to the east. This work will be extended still further over the next two years.

There are now some twenty distribution centres for the Hill Drug Scheme in the Kosi and Mechi zones, all run by local authorities and only checked by the Trust's medical student supervisors. These are British students who, during their final year, have an 'elective period' of three months when they are encouraged to gain experience anywhere in the world, and we take a steady stream of one or two at a time.

The team is now asking for a permanent Director to be

stationed in Kathmandu, as liaison between the Trustees at home and the workers in the field. We are in short ready to operate on a wider basis, supposing that the Nepal Government wishes us to do so; we shall need more long-term and large-scale support for this than we have dared solicit in the past. We have proved ourselves, not only by the calibre of the workers we have been able to recruit, but in the relations we have been able to build up with our colleagues in Nepal.

In short, we have shown that meaningful aid can be offered to a developing country by a very small team, on a very small budget. For less than £30,000 a year we have been able to cover everything: air fares, salaries (all our doctors and nurses are paid the same, nominal, salary), food, housing, porters, transport. This is a great source of pride to us when we think of how wasteful many aid pgojects can be, run by huge administrative staffs, for every penny of our money is spent by our people 'on the ground'.

Today, we get forty or fifty applications for every post we advertise, and we can afford to choose our workers with great care. We need mature and self-reliant young people — early twenties seems to be right — and they must be physically strong (people with very fair skins, for instance, often suffer badly in the heat). And they should be people who want to go for the sheer satisfaction of the work itself, anxious to build something which they may never see complete, and which not they but trained Nepalis in due course will run. We do not, however, propose to expand indefinitely. We see our strength in our small scale, in our lack of full-time administrative offices at home, in our freedom to take immediate decisions on the spot.

And the intimacy of scale has also given a special quality to the relationships we have developed with the country and the people. They are all *working* relationships, based on trust. And in this sense the work of none of us will be lost to the country we set out to assist. In fact, we are all likely to keep our links with the place as close as we can — and many of us indeed will go back, impelled by the consciousness that Nepal is now part of ourselves. When I look around among the early members of the team with whom I am in touch, I am amazed by the extent to which Nepal has become part of our lives.

Barney, who took over as team leader from me in 1971, has already been back to Nepal, as doctor to the Everest Expedition led by Chris Bonnington — he is now back in General Practice in Marlborough, where he and Rachel live with their two small sons. Barney is also Andrew's godfather. Gill has married David, a Ghurkha officer, and they are now in Hong Kong but will certainly see Nepal again. Prue has also married an army officer. Rosemary, on her return to Britain, worked as a Ward Sister in Edinburgh, then went to South Africa, where she married. Peter came back from New Zealand to be accepted as a housefather in a County Council Children's home, one of the youngest people ever to be accepted for such a job. Vint is Senior Registrar in University College Hospital, London, and he and Di live in St Albans with their two children. John also has two children, and he and Sheena live in Kingston where he is Senior Registrar in surgery. Hilary is a District Nurse in Devon, and lecturing on behalf of the Trust. Ann has been training as a Health Visitor, and Jane is a District Nurse in the Shetlands, but since she has done a course in Tropical Medicine in Liverpool, presumably expects to travel again. Peter Fisher (who ran the Hill Drugs Scheme) is in his final medical year at Cambridge and Mark is just behind him at Bristol. Peter Baker has been to the United States, and is now married. Penny and I live in Tonbridge, where I am in General Practice.

And we all hope some day to see Nepal again.

APPENDIX

Some Advice to Travellers

The overland route to the East becomes more popular each year. The following suggestions are made to assist all such would-be travellers.

Allow yourself plenty of time to prepare for the journey. Although technically an easy route, it is hard both on vehicles and drivers and if the vehicle is well equipped much physical and mental strain can be avoided.

Many varieties of vehicle have used this route, from bicycles to buses — I suggest that the landrover is the ideal method of transport; the LWB Wagon affording the most comfort.

I would also suggest that if you can afford it the following extras should be fitted:

2 × 4 gallon water tanks on the front bumpers (never carry petrol here);

2 × 2 gallon Jerricans of Kerosene fixed in cradles beneath the bodywork;

A tropical roof, which gives added comfort; and a small winch is useful. The hydraulic one is very expensive and unnecessary.

Bucket seats in the front are not expensive and well worth incorporating, as is a locking safety compartment under the front centre seat. Seal this off, otherwise it becomes a dust bath.

Everything on the outside of the vehicle should be padlocked — use waterproof locks and try to arrange for all locks to have the same key.

The spare wheel is best mounted on the bonnet and not on the rear door.

The heater can be removed and used as an air cooler — air conditioning is a luxury that few can afford. Fly screens are essential as are European headlights and headlight flashers. A Klaxon horn would be a great advantage.

As for tyres, we used Michelin XYs and found them to be ideal. Two punctures between three vehicles over a combined distance of 24,000 miles speaks for itself. An extra tyre, in addition to the spare wheel, can prove very valuable.

Petrol stations are very frequent and, unless you intend travelling well off the normal routes, the 16-gallon petrol tank is more than adequate. A spare $4\frac{1}{2}$-gallon can however be stored behind the rear seat. Check on petrol prices in each country and fill up before crossing borders to save money.

Carry two gallons of engine oil. It is often expensive and of poor quality in the countries you pass through. After Turkey distilled water is often difficult to obtain and the battery tends to dry out quickly in the hot temperatures.

Spares are difficult to assess but I do advise against the full Rover list, mainly because a spare vehicle would be required to carry it all! I would suggest the following:

4 Inner tubes
Tyre valve replacements
Spare set of wiper blades
Set of plugs
Distributor cap
Set of points
A coil
2 fan-belts
Dynamo
2 oil filters
Glass petrol bulb
Hoses
Set of gaskets

Water pump repair kit
1 set of brake linings
Brake fluid and gear oil

A good set of tools is essêntial; the Rover kit is not sufficient.

Oil, water, battery and tyres should be checked daily and all nuts and bolts tightened at regular intervals. Our exhaust manifolds caused great concern as they continued to rattle loose. These now have locking nuts so future travellers may be spared the luxury of lying on a red hot road, under an even hotter engine, trying to put the exhaust pipe together in one piece.

The A.A. dealt with all our documents most efficiently — international driving licences, green cards and carnets. One book of carnets may not be sufficient so take two, and make certain all details are accurate. The A.A. will help with insurance — third party only is available — and with camping carnets for Europe. I hope that the camping carnet has now been reprinted for it was very inaccurate.

At the time of writing visas are required for Bulgaria, Iran and Afghanistan, all obtainable from the respective Embassies. Allow one day for each visa. Similarly, a border permit is necessary to cross from Pakistan to India at Ferrozapore. This is obtainable either from the Pakistan High Commission in London or en route in Lahore. You may be delayed in Lahore but, on the other hand, if you have no idea of your expected crossing date, a London-issued permit could become out-dated.

Do not overcrowd your vehicle with passengers and if more than one vehicle is involved do not travel in convoy.

Our list of food included the following items:

Milk powder
Tinned meat (stewed steak, spam, etc.)
Vesta meals
Packet soups

Ryvita
Coffee (instant)
Salt
Tinned Butter
Cooking oil or fat
Tinned Sausages
Porridge oats
Tinned fish — tuna, sardines, etc.
Tea
Pepper
Mustard

Medical kit:

Halazone water-sterilising tablets (Boots). Wash all vegetables in halazoned water and after leaving Europe drink only sterilised water however thirsty you are.
Box of elasticised plaster dressings
Cotton wool
Zinc oxide plaster
2 × $\frac{3}{8}'$ Crepe bandages
Aspirin tablets
Sulphaguanidine tablets
Penicillin tablets
Kaolin suspension
Hibitane ointment or Dettol
Insect repellant, suggest DUSK made by Cupal
Caladryl (Calamine plus a local anaesthetic)
Salt tablets
Paludrine (one daily after Turkey as a prophylactic against malaria)
1 pair of scissors
Mycota ointment or powder for athletes foot (Taenia)
Prickly heat powder or ointment
Ear drops — Neocortef
Eye drops — Albucid 10%

Camping is perfectly possible until you reach India. Small

groups are not advised to camp in Northern Persia because of the presence of bandits who might well be tempted to attack. In India, Government rest-houses and 'Dak bungalows' permit privacy and a modicum of comfort.

American dollar travellers' cheques are the best currency — change any Bulgarian money at the frontier before leaving the country; it is not accepted in Turkey. The same applies between Pakistan and India. A very good rate of exchange can be obtained in the Kabul bazaars. Unlimited sterling cheques can be taken for exchange in India. Change money whenever possible at banks and not at the customs posts.

A list of vehicle contents is very useful for Customs purposes with special mention of cameras, radios, etc.

A duplicated letter from your bank is required at certain frontiers to prove that you have the financial means to exist during your stay.

Cholera and smallpox vaccinations are required by International Law. A suggested programme is as follows:

> TABC — Typhoid Paratyphoid — Cholera: 2 injections at 14 days intervals
> TAB should be repeated annually and Cholera at six-month intervals
> Smallpox — 1 injection valid for three years.
> Tetanus — 3 injections, the second and third at six-week and six-month intervals. This gives five years' protection.
> Gamma Globulin 5cc at six-month intervals as a prophylactic against infective hepatitis endemic in Nepal.
> Yellow fever is not required.
> Certificates are only required for smallpox and cholera.

Do not try to do the journey too quickly and you will enjoy it.

Thanks and Acknowledgments

So many people were responsible for the success of our venture that space will not allow me to thank them all. I hope that those I omit will simply know that they helped a worthy project.

My first thanks must go to His late Majesty King Mahendra who gave permission for our team to be established in his country; and to Her Royal Highness Princess Princep Shah who became one of our Patrons and offered us a great deal of sound advice without which we would have been lost in our early days.

Arthur Kellas and all the other members of the British Embassy in Kathmandu were a source of constant strength, clearing paths for us and offering support and personal friendship.

Without belittling the contributions of many hundreds of individuals, and numerous companies and Foundations, I must single out Oxfam and Misereor as our two largest contributors. Oxfam offered help when we were but a name and I hope that they now feel that their support was well judged.

I would like to thank all the members of the Department of Health in Kathmandu together with the many Nepali doctors and nurses who provided us with encouragement and advice, and welcomed us so generously into their country and their homes.

Not least I would like to thank the 'Home team', our

Patrons and Trustees, whose constant support gave us a unique opportunity to establish the firm basis on which others can expand.

Some of the photographs appearing in the book were taken by other members of the team, and I owe them my thanks — as for so much else — for permission to use them. I am also grateful to the Information Service of H.M. Government of Nepal for permission to reproduce illustration 7.